D0064660

The endangered self

To date, the majority of HIV/AIDS research has concentrated on education and prevention for those with a seronegative status, and studies of HIV positive individuals have been concerned with their potential to infect others. *The Endangered Self*, however, focuses on how the discovery of an HIV-positive status affects the individual's sense of identity and on the experience of living with HIV, and its effects on the individual's social relationships.

Drawing upon the concepts of stigma, dangerous identities, and health risk, the authors describe the revaluation that people living with HIV and AIDS must make of the risks entailed by everyday social interactions, and examine their negotiation of these interactions. Chapters discuss issues such as:

- Identity, social risk and AIDS
- Stigma and dangerous identities
- Landscape of risk
- Living and coping with IIIV
- Telling and the danger of disclosure
- Reactions in health care settings and sexual settings
- Risk and reality

In this study, which combines a UK/US perspective, Green and Sobo explore identity change and the stigma attached to an HIV-positive status within the context of the sociology of risk.

Gill Green is a Senior Lecturer at the Health and Social Services Institute, University of Essex. **Elisa J. Sobo** is the Trauma Research Scientist for the Center for Child Health Outcomes, Children's Hospital, San Diego.

HEALTH, RISK AND SOCIETY

Series editor
Graham Hart
MRC Medical Sociology Unit, Glasgow

In recent years, social scientific interest in risk has increased enormously. In the health field, risk is seen as having the potential to bridge the gap between individuals, communities and the larger social structure, with a theoretical framework which unifies concerns around a number of contemporary health issues. This new series will explore the concept of risk in detail, and address some of the most active areas of current health and research practice.

Previous title in this series:

Risk and misfortune
Judith Green

The endangered self
Managing the social risk of HIV

Gill Green and Elisa J. Sobo

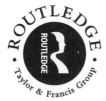

London and New York

First published 2000 in the UK and the USA
by Routledge
11 New Fetter Lane, London EC4P 4EE

Routledge is an imprint of the Taylor & Francis Group

© 2000 Gill Green and Elisa J. Sobo

Typeset in Times by
HWA Text and Data Management, Tunbridge Wells
Printed and bound in Great Britain by
MPG Books Limited, Bodmin

British Library Cataloguing in Publication Data
A catalogue record for this book is available from the British
Library

Library of Congress Cataloging in Publication Data
A catalog record for this book has been requested

ISBN 1-857-28909-9 (hbk)
ISBN 1- 857-28910-2 (pbk)

Contents

Tables

Preface

We are eighteen years into the AIDS epidemic, yet there are relatively few texts which privilege the position of people living with HIV or AIDS, allowing us to see their perspective on the disease. Gill Green and Elisa Sobo, in this second book in the *Health, Risk and Society* series, do precisely that, by giving a voice to those with HIV from such disparate places as North-East England, Scotland's central belt, and New Mexico. The book is also notable because of the wide range of people interviewed in the studies undertaken by the authors. Whether transmission of HIV occurred sexually, through injecting drug use, or through infected blood products (as in those with haemophilia), or whether it is men or women who are speaking, we are fortunate in being granted access to their thoughts and feelings about the experience of being HIV positive. However, the primary strength of the text is its sociological persective on HIV risk. Introducing the concept of 'social risk', Green and Sobo note that social situations always entail risks; "A specifically social risk is a risk ... that might alter one's social relations ... taking a course of action, engaging in a behaviour, or adopting an identity that might alter one's social relations and place in various social networks (e.g. familial, sexual, income-related etc.) and one's position in society as a whole." This permits a more dynamic understanding of the social processes involved in navigating risk landscapes, and in individual and social risk management, than that allowed by the somewhat static concept of stigma (although this remains useful, not least to people with HIV themselves). It also recognises that "taking risks may sometimes have negative outcomes such as rejection, isolation or loss of status," whilst "at other times taking risks may have positive results such as increased support, love and closeness."

Green and Sobo have produced an original and distinctive text rarely seen either in the HIV literature or within the sociology of health and illness. To understand better people's accounts of living with HIV, they employ an analytic framework

PREFACE

and perspective which connects individuals, through daily interactions and experiences in their communities of origin and attachment, to the society in which they live. This book exemplifies the analytic potential of risk and explores fully its many sociological dimensions. I am very pleased indeed to welcome it to the *Health, Risk and Society* series.

Graham Hart
Series Editor
Health, Risk and Society

Acknowledgments

This book is the result of a true partnership between the authors, each of whom contributed equally to this collaborative work. Although the authors jointly accept full responsibility for the content of this volume, data collection for each study described herein was carried out separately. Each author bears responsibility for the integrity of the data from her respective research sites. More importantly, the joint work this book represents could not have been undertaken without the kind help and considered assistance of many individuals and institutions.

The Scottish research was funded by the Medical Research Council of Great Britain and carried out by Gill Green while a member of the MRC Medical Sociology Unit, Glasgow University (Green is now with the Health and Social Services Institute, University of Essex). The work was conducted with Stephen Platt (currently Director of the Research in Health and Behavioural Change Unit in Edinburgh, Scotland); many of the original ideas upon which the study was based were his.

Ruchill Hospital Outpatients and Counselling Clinic, Glasgow Royal Infirmary, Perth and Saughton prisons, Positive Help Edinburgh, the HIV Network in Edinburgh and Body Positive Glasgow kindly allowed the study access to clients. Steven Green, Miriam Guthrie, Helen Mien, Harry Meany, Anne Pinkman, Avril Taylor and Phil Wilson were particularly helpful in facilitating access. Sheena Turner and Stephen Platt conducted many of the interviews, and Mick Bloor, Martin Dunbar, Susan Eley, Graham Hart, Sally Macintyre, Stephen Platt, Patrick West, Danny Wight and Rory Williams provided on-going assistance with the project and helpful comments on resulting papers.

The US research was funded by the Southern Area and Border Health Education Training Centers and by New Mexico State University; the research in England was funded by a Special Project Grant from the University of Durham. The research was undertaken while Sobo was a member of the anthropology departments at

ACKNOWLEDGMENTS

NMSU and UD. In addition to work undertaken there, portions of the analysis of the US data took place at the Center for AIDS Prevention Studies (University of California, San Francisco), and the final synthesis was carried out at the University of California, San Diego.

Paula Black, Jude Drapeau, and Michelle Nawrocki provided invaluable research assistance for Sobo's projects. AIDS service workers Dorothy Ball, Terry Call, Paul Court, Megan McGuire, Jim McManus, David Miller, Lizzy Pearce, Pat Ramshaw, David Simonsmeier, Carl Valles, Debbie Wiltshire, Gail Wheeler and others provided crucial support by endorsing the projects, discussing them with clients and colleagues, and otherwise providing assistance with recruitment outreach. Institutions providing recruitment support in England included Body Positive North East Limited, Cleveland AIDS Support, the GUM (STD) unit at Dreyburn Hospital in Durham, the Family Unit at Middlesbrough General Hospital, Northern Counties Trust for People Living with AIDS, and MESMAC (Men who have Sex with Men Action in the Community). In New Mexico, recruitment and staging assistance was provided through Sun Country Case Management and Southwest AIDS Committee. F.G. Bailey, Frederick Bloom, Peter Collins, Victor de Munck, Thomas Hall, Michael Herzfeld, Sushrut Jadhav, Nina Kammerer, Peter Keogh, Murray Last, Roland Littlewood, Cheryl Rock, Scott Rushforth, Harvey Smallman, and Donald Tuzin kindly offered comments or other generous forms of support that helped bring this project to fruition.

Charlie Davison, Simon Carter and Graham Hart provided the impetus and invaluable assistance to set the entire study within the context of the sociology of risk: we draw heavily upon Davison's concept of 'landscapes of risk', and Carter's work linking risk with identity, and it was Hart who suggested we interpret our data from a risk perspective.

Thanks are also due to the Sociology Department, University of Essex, which provided funds enabling the authors to meet to develop this joint work.

While this book puts forth an original argument, portions of the data presented here have been described previously, and several papers previously published have been drawn or quoted from to support the present analysis. The publishers of these articles have kindly granted us permission to reproduce or otherwise draw from selected extracts for this book as needed. They are: Taylor & Francis, Blackwell Publishers (*Sociology of Health and Illness*), Pergamon (*Social Science and Medicine*), Sage Publications (*Journal of Health Psychology*), Carfax (*Anthropology & Medicine*), and University of Pennsylvania Press. Stephen Platt, who co-authored a number of articles with Green, also has granted his kind permission to reprint segments from work he jointly penned.

ACKNOWLEDGMENTS

We are grateful to all of the individuals and institutions associated with this project. But greatest thanks go to the research participants in Scotland, England, and the USA, without whom this work would not have been possible and to whom our effort here is dedicated. Each graciously contributed time and effort to this project, selflessly sharing with us intimate aspects of their private experiences in order to help us to fill the great gaps in our knowledge on the links between risk, stigma, and identity. We have altered superficial details in some of their stories in order to ensure anonymity, and use only pseudonyms. It is our hope that participants will agree that we have aptly captured their opinions and compellingly conveyed some sense of what it is to be – in one's own eyes or others', and in ways that shift with every flux in social context – a person with AIDS or HIV.

About the Authors

Gill Green is a medical sociologist based at the Health and Social Services Institute, University of Essex. Her research in the field of HIV began in 1990 at the MRC Medical Sociology Unit at Glasgow and has resulted in numerous published articles, e.g. 'Fear and loathing in health care settings reported by people with HIV', *Sociology of Health and Illness* (1997); 'Now and again it really hits you: the impact of an HIV diagnosis upon psycho-social well-being,' *Journal of Health Psychology* (1996); 'Attitudes towards people with HIV: are they as stigmatizing as people with HIV think they are?', *Social Science and Medicine* (1995). She is currently continuing her research about the experience of chronic illness with a study of social risk and identity among people with severe mental illness. Green is also is involved in a number of other collaborative applied research projects with the North East Essex Mental Health Trust and North Essex Health Authority. Her research on HIV/AIDS now focuses on areas of the developing world, specifically Uganda, where the disease remains rampant.

Elisa J. Sobo is a medical anthropologist based in the Center for Child Health Outcomes at Children's Hospital of San Diego. Her interest in HIV/AIDS developed as a result of her work on Caribbean health traditions. In addition to continuing research on sexual and reproductive health, Sobo is involved in childhood injury prevention and control research, as well as the Olestra Post-Marketing Surveillance Study, a national (USA) nutrition-related project, where her focus is on child-centred data-collection methods. As an editorial board member for *Anthropology & Medicine*, Sobo has assembled and edited two special issues, including one on

ACKNOWLEDGMENTS

HIV/AIDS (Volume 6, Number 1). Publications include: *Choosing Unsafe Sex: AIDS Risk Denial and Disadvantaged Women* (University of Pennsylvania Press 1995); *One Blood: The Jamaican Body* (SUNY 1993); *The Cultural Context of Health, Illness, and Medicine* (Bergin & Garvey 1997, co-authored with M. Loustaunau); and *Using Methods in the Field: a Practical Introduction and Casebook* (AltaMira/Sage 1998, with V. de Munck). Co-edited collections on contraception (Berg) and celibacy (University of Wisconsin Press) are forthcoming.

Chapter 1

Identity, social risk, and AIDS: what's the connection?

Introduction

Acquired Immune Deficiency Syndrome (AIDS), the disease state brought on by infection with Human Immunodeficiency Virus (HIV), took the world by surprise in the early 1980s. When the US Centers for Disease Control and Prevention (CDC), which first defined the syndrome, began surveillance practices in 1982, they counted 248 cases (Walker 1991). But it very soon became clear that these few US cases represented the tip of a growing global iceberg. Just over 10 years later, about 3 million people world-wide had died of AIDS; about 15 million people were infected with HIV (WHO 1994). Fifteen years later, at the end of 1997, 30.6 million individuals around the world were living with HIV or AIDS. AIDS had taken the lives of 11.7 million people, leaving 8.2 million children as orphans. In 1997 alone, 5.8 million new HIV infections were diagnosed (WHO 1998: 5).

While a by far larger proportion of those infected or killed by the virus and its complications live in less developed nations such as those in Africa and Asia than in the UK or the USA, the effects of the virus in the latter nations still has been staggering. In the UK, by the end of September 1998, 32,925 people had been diagnosed with HIV and 17,777 with AIDS (PHLS AIDS Centre 1998). In the USA, according to CDC estimates, perhaps 750,000 people were infected with HIV by the early 90s (McQuillan et al. 1994). By 1998, over half a million US residents had been diagnosed with AIDS and the accepted HIV infection estimate had risen to one million (Kalichman and Fisher 1998: 87).

Health is a social process and, as is the case world-wide, HIV is not uniformly distributed throughout US and UK populations. It penetrates social networks so that the likelihood of infection is highest among gay men and impoverished people of colour living in the pandemic's urban epicentres.

The threat of HIV infection, and of AIDS, has generated many responses, some hysterical, some level-headed, and some apathetic. This book represents the combined efforts of a medical sociologist (Green) and a medical anthropologist (Sobo) to document and examine the varied responses to AIDS and to HIV of three groups of HIV-positive UK and US individuals. We focus specifically on the social risks HIV infection entails, the ways in which those risks are internalized in relation to identity construction, and the manner by which they are confronted in the everyday lives of people with HIV or AIDS.

Present goals

Understanding the everyday experiences of people with HIV or AIDS is a crucial step in reducing the human costs of the pandemic. To date, the majority of published HIV/AIDS research in the social sciences concerns education and prevention among the seronegative (some reviews and collections include Bolton and Singer 1992b; Coyle *et al.* 1991; Rotheram-Borus *et al.* 1995).

There is, however, an emerging social scientific literature concerned with life after infection with HIV (e.g. Adam and Sears 1996; Cowles and Rodgers 1997; Crossley 1997; Davies 1997; McCain and Gramling 1992; Ward 1993a; Siegel and Krauss 1991). The growth of this literature notwithstanding, few authors have attended to HIV specifically in relation to identity processes, such as the ongoing crafting, negotiation and redefinition of context-specific selves (e.g. as described in Sandstrom 1990; see also Hassin 1994; Rymes 1995). A positive HIV antibody test can shatter a previously crafted sense of self, and it can mean that an individual will incorporate a new facet into his or her identity – that of being HIV positive. HIV can be a secret identity factor or one publicly proclaimed. And for some, it may not figure at all: some may ignore, reject, or otherwise not incorporate their HIV serostatus into their identities.

The manner in which chronic illness interacts with and moulds identity has received attention (see Bury 1982, 1991; Charmaz 1987; Corbin and Strauss 1988; Herzlich and Pierret 1987; Scambler and Hopkins 1986) but the processes involved in refashioning or adjusting one's identity to reflect testing positive for HIV and the ways in which a positive test can affect life experience have only begun to come under scrutiny (e.g. Ariss with Dowsett 1997; Gatter 1995). Our analysis of identity-formation and manipulation among the HIV positive can shed further light on these processes, and it can do so in a way that advances social-scientific theory related to risk. We believe that HIV/AIDS identity-linked processes are, in fact, best understood when potential HIV-related alterations in the risk landscape the individual occupies are taken into account. We are especially interested in the social risks that HIV seropositivity entail. That is, although HIV/AIDS is a physical health issue, we are interested in risks that are primarily social rather than organic or biological.

Social risk may vary with social factors such as class, gender, ethnicity and age. Nevertheless, certain aspects of the economically developed world's response to HIV/AIDS are similar across populations, so in some respects the social risk of being HIV positive are similar for most people in such countries. Our work explores these similarities and differences.

There exists a rich literature on stigma, and the socio-cultural construction and management of dangerous identities (traceable to Goffman 1963; e.g. Jones *et al.* 1984; regarding AIDS stigma *per se*, see Sandstrom 1990; Siegel and Krauss 1991; Alonzo and Reynolds 1995). Current interest in the sociology of risk (e.g. Beck 1992; Giddens 1991; Gabe 1995) and the anthropology of the same (e.g. Douglas 1985, 1982; Bellaby 1990) does exist. Notwithstanding, very little has been written about social risk in relation to health in general and stigmatized health conditions in particular. Many studies of health risk, especially those relating to HIV, have instead focused upon behaviour specifically associated with negative health outcomes (e.g. condomless penetrative sex, which may lead to infection, or crossinfection, or the infection of others, with HIV). People's revaluation of the risks entailed by everyday social interactions after diagnosis with terminal or chronic disease conditions and their negotiation of these interactions have not received much attention (some exceptions are Gordon 1990; Murphy 1998; Bury 1991). Our work seeks to help fill this gap in the health-related risk literature in general and especially in the literature on HIV/AIDS. We attempt to help answer Hart and Boulton's call for a 'sociology of risk' (1995) by highlighting the social and cultural factors that influence risk perception among HIV-positive people as well as risk-related decision making.

A fuller understanding of the subjective, lived experience of having one's health threatened by a chronic, stigmatized, identity-transforming disease can be had through the development of an advanced sociology of risk – one that incorporates key theoretical concepts from the fields of stigma management, identity construction and risk. To this end, we explore the context-dependent processes whereby a person with HIV determines the extent to which his or her seropositivity is a source of danger or difference and we investigate the processes underlying the partial or complete identification one may make with one's endangered or endangering self. We examine the ways in which the risk landscape may shift in relation to an HIV-transformed social identity as well as the ways in which risk management strategies related to this shift are devised, assimilated into, and expressed in, social interactions. We take as our focus the processual relationship between culturally conditioned risk perception, social interaction and identity maintenance and (re)formation.

While HIV infection and AIDS are different conditions, they are both part of the same disease continuum; AIDS results from infection with HIV. Further, the line between the two terms when used to describe socially and culturally constructed symbolic domains is very blurry indeed. For this reason, and for verbal efficiency in the text, we will generally speak of both conditions uniformly from hereon. Unless a distinction needs to be made for contextualizing purposes, we will refer to people living with HIV or AIDS as 'PHAs', and when talking about HIV/AIDS, we will generally use only one acronym or the other. Because much public discourse regarding HIV/AIDS centres more overtly around AIDS than HIV, when speaking about public perceptions the term 'AIDS' will generally be used. On the other hand, when speaking about the people who participated in the research, unless the fact that a person has AIDS *per se* is relevant to the discussion, we use the term 'HIV positive', because it is more inclusive.

Future possibilities

We are writing this book at what is currently perceived to be a crucial juncture in the natural history of AIDS: we are now witnessing increases in quality of life and improved survival statistics for those in wealthier nations with access to leading-edge medical care. In the UK, deaths from AIDS have fallen dramatically each quarter since 1997 and in the second and third quarters of 1998 numbered less than 50. This figure is significantly lower than the 200–400 reported each quarter from 1990 to 1995 (PHLS AIDS Centre 1998). In the USA, yearly AIDS death rates began to fall in 1996. While in 1995, deaths numbered 49,985, in 1996 they numbered just 37,525. And in 1997, they decreased 42 per cent again, to 21,909 (CDC 1998: 36). The decrease was greater among men (44%) than women (32%), and greater among whites (51%) (CDC 1998: 3).[1] It is clear that people with HIV or AIDS who have access to the new combination therapies and protease inhibitors are living longer and more productive lives than they previously would have believed

4

possible. Whilst it is not known how long the therapeutic drugs will outpace the progression of the virus, the fall in death rate has renewed optimism.

But as the breakdown of the US decrease figures suggest, advanced therapies are not available on an equal basis to all. Further, world-wide, the AIDS toll continues to grow at an alarming pace (Singer 1999). This and the benefits of unexpected survival notwithstanding, the shock of finding oneself alive and well when one expected to be long dead or at least disabled may lead to many complications – complications that we cannot directly address in this book but which are anticipated in our data. They were anticipated directly by at least some HIV-positive people to whom we spoke, although we never asked about them. In a 1996 discussion about the way that HIV has altered his approach to daily life, Joe Watson[2] (to whom you will later be formally introduced) told us:

> Somebody said to me in the group I go to, "If they found a miracle cure would you want it?" I said "I don't think I would now." I've got so used to – I've gone through so much heart ache, so much crying, pulling my hair out. ...I've got so used to the way I am now and my outlook on life and what life's got left of it I think I'd – I wouldn't want it, it would be too much of an upheaval again and I don't want to go through all that worry and stress and I don't think I'd want it. I know where I am now.

There can be no doubt that the experience of displacement, reorientation and confrontation with AIDS-related social risks that we write about in this book, and that Joe describes as an "upheaval," will have an impact on survivors' lives. Our conclusions, therefore, may have implications not only for PHAs in the early and middle 1990s, when our research was conducted, nor just for those without access to breakthrough therapies (and the majority of PHAs world-wide will remain in this category well into the twenty-first century), but also for those who will be lucky enough to reduce their viral loads and increase their life expectancies. The experiences that we describe may hold clues or predictive value relevant to the experiences of this group too. We hope, then, that research related not only to the topic at hand but also that which relates to long term survival may find much to build on in the findings presented here.

The structure of the volume

We, the authors, Sobo and Green, joined forces in 1996. This pairing was based on common research interests, regional proximity, and a realization of striking similarities between our disparately collected findings. While data collection and primary analyses were carried out separately, secondary analyses and the related contextualizing literature, research and synthetic work represented in this volume were carried out conjointly and with unified intent.

With this book, we seek to display the whole picture our AIDS research reveals, using narratives of PHAs as the primary data source. In the findings sections, the PHAs speak for themselves, inasmuch as this is possible, while we highlight common themes and the social and cultural mechanisms that underlie their stories. Only when people's stories are presented within an analytic context can we hope to provide in full the services and support that PHAs require if they are to prosper or at least survive socially in the face of the devastating, deadly physical effects of AIDS.

In this introductory chapter, we set out the major concepts to be explored: stigma, identity, social risk, and risk landscape. While Chapters 2 and 3 review the literature, identify gaps in our knowledge, and define the parameters of our investigation, we do not limit our discussion of previous research to the 'front part' of the volume. Throughout the book, we cycle back and forth between our findings and the literature, building support for our position in a spiraling fashion; we return as needed to topics earlier introduced and expand our discussion of them as our argument builds and insights grow.[3] Notwithstanding, most of the foundations for our presentation of data are laid in these two chapters.

In Chapter 2, we investigate the stigmatization process in relation to AIDS, and examine the cultural construction of the seropositive person. HIV infection is seen as something that happens to particular types of people in particular circumstances and these understandings underwrite variation in the ways that people of different backgrounds, and with different relationships to the factors thought to be linked with HIV infection, experience being associated with AIDS. Variations notwithstanding, association with AIDS is risky because of its negative connotations. Readers are introduced to the processes entailed in crafting – or rejecting – a potentially dangerous and thereby risky identity that incorporates a positive HIV serostatus, as well as the social process of story-telling through which such identities are given currency.

Social situations always entail risks; a specifically social risk is one that can lead to a change in one's social standing and esteem. While specific actions can be risky, having a certain type of identity – for example, one that is negatively stigmatized –

also can be risky. In Chapter 3 we explain how knowledge that one has a socially risky identity affects one's approach to social situations; it affects one's navigation of what we refer to (after Davison 1991b) as the 'risk landscape'. We explore the ramifications that being ascribed and internalizing – in full or just in part – a spoiled or dangerous identity can have for navigating this landscape. We also question taken-for-granted definitions of risk. The subjective and the socio-culturally organized aspects of risk are discussed, and the role that the increased consciousness we have of risk in today's world may play in PHAs' social risk management strategies is examined. We pay special attention to the perceived dangers of disclosure – dangers that we contend are in some ways exaggerated due to cultural and social factors related to the stigmatization of AIDS.

Chapter 4 describes the various settings and methods for the research that spurred this book. While the largest segment of data collection was conducted in Scotland, other research took place in North-East England and in New Mexico, USA. This chapter explains the particulars of each project and describes the framework for the integration of the findings.

Chapter 5 examines the process of testing positive and the consequences for mental and physical health. Our findings regarding post-test psycho-social well-being are discussed. We then examine the socio-cultural construction of spoiled and dangerous identities that arise as a consequence of testing positive. The various culturally defined aspects of identity that can be affected by the incorporation of serostatus information are discussed, as is the whole process of internalizing or rejecting a newly available identity component.

One of the primary concerns of the chronically ill revolves around the issue of social support and assistance. Chapters 6 and 7 examine the processes whereby PHAs decide whether to retain an HIV identity (or identity facet) as private knowledge or whether to disclose it. The various reasons for each position are examined, as are reported outcomes of voluntarily revealing one's positive serostatus and of nonvoluntarily having it revealed.

Self-disclosure generally is necessary for garnering social support specifically related to AIDS. Various patterns of disclosure are examined and the cultural understandings or social factors underlying them, such as understandings related to responsibility or constructions of social distance. Benefits and dangers of self-disclosure are scrutinized in relation to the various social risks such disclosure entails. In light of what will be, for many an HIV-positive person, perceived as a drastically altered landscape of risk, various strategies for risk assessment and self-disclosure exist. The delicate processes entailed in making such assessments and acting on decisions are examined, and we discuss the ways such decisions articulate with cultural expectations for friends and family.

Chapters 8, 9 and 10 further examine disclosure issues, specifically concentrating on reported outcomes in, and expectations for, self-disclosure in settings where relations are more physically intimate than they may be amongst family and friends. Chapter 8 concentrates on disclosure in health care settings; Chapters 9 and 10 examine the particular case of disclosure in the intimate arena of conjugal or sexual relations, where HIV transmission is most likely.

In public settings, such as health centres, discrimination and breaches of confidentiality are major concerns and when they come from health care workers, who are supposed to be objective and nonjudgmental, they may be particularly damaging to self-concept. In the conjugal or sexual arena, fears of rejection are paramount. Public opprobrium related to fear of infection has led in some locations to the criminalization of certain sexual practices when engaged in by PHAs, and persons found guilty of engaging in outlawed actions can pay heavy penalties. Notwithstanding, the response from sexual partners may in general be supportive, and it may be better than the response from professional caregivers. PHAs' decisions about whether to have sex (and, if so, of what type), whether to have committed sexual relationships, and whether to have children are investigated, as are the cultural ideals for relationships that may motivate such decisions. The process of balancing the risks entailed in each of these decisions is examined in detail.

Chapter 11 examines social contacts' response to disclosure with reference to statistical, quantitative data. Differences in the general experiences of groups of people with HIV are examined; we are especially interested in the impacts of socio-cultural factors, such as those related to gender, ethnicity, social class, sexual orientation, drug use, and prior experience of illness. As in the previous chapters, the extent to which PHAs' perceptions of disclosure's risks equate with their actual experience of negative responses following disclosure is discussed. Our data indicate that the match is problematic: PHAs tend to overestimate the hostility of others towards them. The reported responses and the expected responses differed significantly, and the perception that social networks will shrink on disclosure was not supported by empirical data. Discussion sheds light upon the relationship between risk perception and lived experience.

In Chapter 12, we review the significance of stigma and social risk for the creation and maintenance of certain kinds of identities and certain levels of social well being. Variations in the presentation of the endangered self in society, noted throughout the preceding chapters, are explored as part of our summarizing efforts, with particular reference to variation in the landscape of risk. We show how presentation of the endangered self varies according to social context. A PHA may in some contexts embrace an HIV identity whilst rejecting it at other times or in

8

other social contexts. The range of identities and risk management strategies adopted by people with HIV are linked to such differences.

Our research suggests that, despite variation, people with HIV share an elevated perception of social risk. This can only be understood when the special risk landscapes of people with chronic illness and individuals with stigmatized or dangerous identities are taken into account. Routine social action that for the HIV-negative and untested would not even be linked consciously with the notion of risk may, for the HIV-positive, bring that notion to the forefront of consciousness. The ramifications of our data for service providers, educators, and researchers as well as in relation to the service entitlements and social rights and needs of PHAs are discussed. Identity construction is linked to a more general understanding of social risk management as a critical feature of everyday life in society, for people with HIV or AIDS and for people without it.

Notes

1   The incidence of AIDS also is on the decrease; between 1996 and 1997, the incidence in the USA decreased 15 per cent overall. Decreases were smaller for women than men, and smaller for Blacks and among those with heterosexual infections (CDC 1998: 3).
2   All names given are pseudonyms. In addition, we avoid mention of, or slightly alter, potentially identifying details to protect participant anonymity. We do so only where omission or slight alteration does not affect the discussion regarding the data being presented. Joe is a member of the sample of PHAs from the North-East of England.
3   This technique is modeled on the methods of hermeneutics and grounded theory.

Chapter 2

Dangerous identities: stigmas and stories

The subjective side of AIDS[1]

Most research carried out with people with HIV or AIDS (PHAs) considers them as the objects of study (Adam and Sears 1994). PHAs (or: their body parts and systems) are studied as specimens by medical research specialists who seek to help limit the damage HIV can do. Epidemiologists sort seropositive people into risk groups, the swelling and shrinking of which is observed and interpreted. Cultural and social theorists also objectify PHAs as, for example, in investigations of the processes of signification, cultural construction, marginalization and social cohesion. In such studies, PHAs are taken as signs to be read or strategically deployed.

The latter form of research has led to a number of exceptional critiques of contemporary culture and socio-political organization, some of which we draw upon in this book. But while scholarly attention has been lavished on the PHAs' seropositive body as a symbol, the actual experiences of the HIV-positive person in the face of what Treichler in 1987 titled the "epidemic of signification" has received less attention, at least in the academic literature (some exceptions are Adam and Sears 1994; Adam and Sears 1996; Crossley 1997; Davies 1997; Carricaburu and Pierret 1995; Lang 1991).[2]

This is not to say that we have no idea about the self-reported frequencies of certain actions or feelings of PHAs. The literature is full of figures denoting how many people with HIV do what and with whom and how often (at least so far as sex, drug use, and care-related actions go). But the complex subjective (and intersubjective) reasons motivating the numbers reported often remain unexamined or taken for granted.

The need for an experience-near or process-centred approach that "explores the *subjectivity* of AIDS" (Adam and Sears 1994: 63; emphasis in text) is especially clear in the area of stigma research and related efforts to examine the social risks that seropositivity entails. As Adam and Sears note, in regard to self-disclosure *per se*, most of what little we know is confined to quantitative data from urban US gay men.[3]

There are publications that examine what it is like to be HIV positive. However, only recently have such publications come out of academic endeavours (e.g. Ariss with Dowsett 1997; Cajetan Luna 1997; Klitzman 1997). Further, even legitimate academic publications on the topic are not scholarly treatises in the usual sense. They often fail to contextualize the subjective, self-reported beliefs or experiences of the HIV-positive people that they present and provide little in the way of objective analysis or quantitative verification or corroboration. Rather, they tend to take as self-evident the claims of discrimination, related social losses and a resulting shrinking of the social networks of PHAs.

In their discussion of suffering as social experience, Kleinman and Kleinman explain that "modes of suffering" or "patterns of how to undergo troubles ... are taught and learned, sometimes openly, often indirectly" (1996: 2). PHAs' claims of social loss after testing positive for HIV may be readily accepted because they fit so well with the beliefs many people hold about the stigma attached to AIDS. They fit with the models commonly put forth about what is supposed to happen upon receiving a positive diagnosis: the cultural mode of suffering ascribed to AIDS. Reluctance to question these claims also may stem from the political incorrectness of stating that having AIDS is not necessarily as socially destructive as it is reputed to be. This is not to deny the horrible nature of the disease but rather to point out that in certain respects the disease may be more benign socially than is commonly believed.

Kleinman and Kleinman show that cultural preparation for certain modes of suffering "far too often are part of the problem; they become iatrogenic" (1996: 9). While the Kleinmans were referring specifically to public complacency regarding forms of suffering they have come to take for granted, we can extend their argument to those enduring the suffering. Thus, we contend that as a result of a belief in social alienation arising from a positive diagnosis, PHAs may choose not to disclose their serostatus or request support from family, friends, care providers, or lovers. In other words, they may deny themselves support that might be forthcoming simply because they believe that it will not. Accordingly, disclosure to, and the support from, such classes of people is a central topic in this book.

In an effort to add to our understanding of what it means to have a 'dangerous identity', such as being HIV positive, in this book we explore the process of self-disclosing that one is seropositive. We focus upon the process of 'telling'and we do so, in as much as it is possible, from the PHAs' point of view. Discussing telling not only entails examining seropositivity disclosure *per se*, but also involves examining the factors that block disclosure as well as those that enable it. It entails a full exploration of the social and cultural context in which disclosure of being HIV positive does and does not happen. It involves a full examination of the social risk of 'owning' an HIV identity as well as an examination of the practical ramifications of these risks. Through these investigations, we hope to augment knowledge about HIV's devastating physical consequences, which must never be trivialized or forgotten, with increased understanding of some of the social and cultural aspects of various other subjectively experienced ramifications of infection with HIV.

Rather than attempting to describe what PHAs actually do, our work for the most part explores how they talk about what they do. By examining stigma management and self-disclosure from this angle, we hope to avoid the easily-made mistake of equating what people say they do with what they do in practice. Notwithstanding, we do have some quantitative data that deals with actual practice, and later we present it in order to provide a fuller picture of the PHAs' experience.

In examining narrative or story-telling practices, and the stories told, we hope to shed some light on the intersubjective processes of stigma management and on the (almost) never-ending process of identity formulation (*cf.* Gatter 1995; Hassin 1994; Rymes 1995). By investigating the objective reality of some of the stories told, we hope to shed further light on the experience of what we call 'endangered selfhood'. But before we look to these processes and products, let us discuss what it means to bear a stigma and to navigate a landscape of social risk.

What is stigma?

Basic definitions

Knowledge that AIDS carries a stigma is commonplace, at least among liberals and others who would defend people infected with it. But the term 'stigma' is offered up, even in academic literature, as if its meaning is understood by all. That is, its meaning – and the meaning of the 'AIDS = stigma' equation – generally is left unsaid. What, exactly, does the blanket term 'stigma' cover? How does stigma manage to mark people? And why are we so afraid of it?

The modern term 'stigma' stems from a Latin word describing a prick with a pointed instrument. A stigma is, literally, "a distinguishing mark burned or cut into the flesh, as of a slave or criminal," serving most typically as a "mark of disgrace or reproach" (Webster 1983: 1788). Beside physical marks, nonphysical characteristics, too, such as spinsterhood, can serve as stigmata (stigma's plural). In either case, an individual's failure to live up to social and cultural ideals is highlighted, whether by a physical blemish or by a state of being – an identity (or a facet thereof). Indeed, the spoiling process associated with stigma may eclipse a person's social identity so that s/he is treated as belonging to a stigmatized category (e.g. as a 'cripple', a 'drunk', a 'paedophile') rather than as an individual, and devalued in the process (Zola 1993).

Stigma has, in certain historical settings, carried positive meaning: "For Christians, stigmatic markings could signify special grace" (Herek 1990: 109). Notwithstanding, modern social science deems stigma a negative construct. Our knowledge of stigma's roots in failure to fulfill one's ascribed role stems largely from Erving Goffman's widely-cited book, *Stigma: notes on the management of spoiled identity*, the 1963 publication of which established the study of stigma as a valid academic pursuit.

"By definition," Goffman wrote, "we believe the person with a stigma is not quite human" (1963: 15). Goffman cast stigma as a socially constructed deviance label. Therefore, what is stigmatizing in one place and time may not be so in another. In other words, stigma is a culturally relative construction.

Moreover, stigma as Goffman (1963) describes it is not an essential feature of an attribute like, say, a visible physical deformity or a deviant act, but rather it emerges as a result of social reactions to such attributes. Stigma is a social product generated by social interactions in which potentially stigmatizing attributes (or unrealized norms) are relevant to either party's expectations. Writes Goffman (1963: 137–138):

> Stigma involves not so much a set of concrete individuals who can be separated into two piles, the stigmatized and the normal, as a pervasive two-role social process in which every individual participates in both roles. ...The normal and the stigmatized are not persons but rather perspectives.

The impact of stigma in everyday life is thus related to its inherently social nature; every day, discrediting associations are made during the stigmatized individual's social interactions, whether imagined and anticipated, or experienced for real.

Facets of stigma

Stigmata vary along numerous dimensions, including degree of disruptiveness, aesthetics or aesthetic qualities, cause or origin, course or changes over time, the degree of peril held for others, and concealability (Jones *et al.* 1984; see also Herek 1990). Summing up the literature, Crandall and Moriarty write, "The disruptiveness dimension is clearly important in determining the extent to which a particular stigma interferes with a person's everyday life" (1995: 68).

Disruptiveness, aesthetics and concealability are affected by, among other things, the degree to which stigmata are obvious and external, as would be the case with visible lesions, as opposed to those which are hidden, internal, or ideational, so that one 'can't tell by looking'. People with visible stigmata such as severe burns, dwarfism, or acute neurofibramatosis (thought to have afflicted the so-called 'Elephant Man') face potential disruption from all people in their social milieu (see Knudson-Cooper 1981; Ablon 1981, 1995). Clearly, information control becomes a central concern for people with hidden stigmata that may, if revealed, become highly disruptive.

Goffman (1963) draws a useful distinction between being 'discreditable' (possessing a hidden stigma and not disclosing it) and being 'discredited' (possessing a visible stigma or having disclosed or been found by others to have a heretofore hidden one). People with hidden stigmata, which in our culture include such things as undisclosed criminal records or mental illness, are discreditable. The discreditable are able to disclaim socially their possession of a stigmatizing attribute and may tell nobody or only those they want to know about the situation. However, they have to live with the possibility that people may accidentally (or through malicious gossip) find out about the stigmatizing attribute, which will thereby become discrediting.

Other key dimensions of stigma, at least in relation to physical illness, are origin, course and peril. Crandall and Moriarty cite a number of studies finding that the "first dimension in disease representation was onset controllability" (1995: 69). Onset controllability – the degree to which a disease is preventable – is correlated with social rejection not only in studies they cite but also in their own work (more of which later).

14

Diseases or disabilities that become more pronounced over time, such as HIV when it becomes symptomatic and more overtly discrediting, are also associated with more negative societal reactions. So too are illnesses that are contagious and thus associated with peril.

Internalization and identity

Distaste for the stigmatized does not only come from those who are 'normal'. Goffman (1963) has described how stigmatized persons who would be part of the social group that abhors their stigma will incorporate and internalize the often harsh cultural standards for perfection held by that wider society of which they too are a part, and thereby discredit themselves. Self-hatred and shame develop from internalizing a negative valuation of one's self or body. The discrepancy between what is expected in a normal individual and what is actual in a stigmatized individual 'spoils' the social identity (the culturally conditioned identity that is important in social interactions), and limits the level of social acceptance s/he might expect (Alonzo and Reynolds 1995). Negative cultural attitudes held by members of the mainstream, core, or (in other words) dominant culture towards stigmatized people are thus important sources of internalized stigma, and serve to pattern the individual's self-conception in a self-fulfilling manner (Williams 1987).

The individual's stigma can come to dominate both his or her own and others' perceptions, and achieve what Hughes (1945) called "master-status," that according to Schneider and Conrad (1981: 217) "'floods' one's identity and life with meanings and behaviour that figuratively constipate the social self." Whilst such a swamping may generally be a negative process, many people have used the concept of master-status to form powerful self-help groups to further their rights to achieve political goals (see Zola 1993), or to develop acceptance of a new self-identity (see Ablon 1981). Some PHAs have asserted a positive identity in this manner, e.g. activists who discover a newfound purpose and identity through AIDS.

Another way of talking about variance along the internalization dimension is to discuss stigma as either 'felt' or 'enacted'. This distinction was first recognized among people with epilepsy (Scambler and Hopkins 1986). Enacted stigma refers to a situation in which sanctions are individually or collectively applied to people with a condition, while felt stigma relates to feelings of shame and an oppressive fear engendered by the spectre of enacted stigma. Shame is a key word here: felt stigma involves not just anticipation of bias but internalization of it as well.

A person with a high degree of felt stigma may tend to blame negative occurrences or reactions on his or her stigma *per se*, rather than see others as intolerant.

For example, Crocker *et al.* (1993) found that overweight female psychology under-graduates tended to attribute negative dating-related feedback to their weight rather than to see their dates as biased against fat people. The distinction between blaming one's stigma and blaming an evaluator's prejudice is subtle, but important: "Attribu-tions to the stigma itself that are not associated with attributions to prejudice do not externalize negative feedback or outcomes" (p. 62). Rather, they internalize these, associating them with the stigmatized self.

External attributions may be less damaging. Indeed, many studies demonstrate the self-protective function of this coping strategy. In their literature review, Crocker *et al.* (1993) cite studies showing that women who attribute negative evaluations to prejudice have higher self-esteem and are lower in depressed affect than those who do not. Another study showed that negatively evaluated Black students who know their evaluators can see them (compared to those who know that they cannot be seen by evaluators) do not experience a decrease in self-esteem as they can blame a negative evaluation on the evaluator's assumed prejudice against darker-skinned people.[4] Stigma in this case provides a ready, externalizing explanation for negative outcomes or feedback, thus protecting self-esteem and mood (Crocker *et al.* 1991, as cited in Crocker *et al.* 1993: 61). But when stigma is 'felt' and internalized, it may not be so easily drawn on in service of one's social or affective well being.

Both felt and enacted stigma may have severe social consequences for individuals in terms of their rights, freedom, self-identity and social interactions, and both may have psychopathological consequences (Arnston 1986; Jacoby 1994). In Scambler and Hopkins' (1986) aforementioned study of epilepsy, people experienced felt stigma before, and whether or not, they experienced enacted stigma. Felt stigma was more prevalent than enacted, and it predisposed the stigmatized to conceal their condition to protect against experiencing enacted discrimination and prejudice.

In a study building on these findings, Jacoby (1994) found that, among people with epilepsy in the UK, the frequency of self-reported social activity in the three months prior to participation in the study was not related to felt stigma. However, felt stigma scores and the perception that social activities were restricted because of epilepsy (whether or not they were) were significantly and positively correlated. Further, although employment rates of the sample and the UK population were similar, one-third of the sample felt that epilepsy did make it more difficult for them than other people to secure work. Later chapters examine the possibility that similarly skewed feelings of social restriction and discrimination may be present among PHAs.

The stigmatizing nature of AIDS

The double deviance of PHAs

Notwithstanding the important advances in treatment that may have transformed HIV for some from a terminal into a chronic illness, seropositivity remains one of the most stigmatized and stigmatizing health conditions known. The negative valuation of AIDS and its negative symbolic connotations are to a large extent the result of cultural processes whereby boundaries are drawn between the 'healthy self' and the 'unhealthy other' who is imagined as contagious, sexually deviant and addicted (Crawford 1994). PHAs are stigmatized because AIDS is viewed as the responsibility of the individual, perceived as contagious, not well understood by health care providers, and associated with an unaesthetic and undesirable death (Alonzo and Reynolds 1995).

Whilst death, contagion, unhealthy 'otherness', and personal culpability may be associated with many illnesses, the fact that AIDS has been most prevalent in Europe and North America among gay men and drug users who were already targets of prejudice (Herek and Glunt 1989) has meant that PHAs are linked with so-called 'deviant' behaviour. PHAs living in these regions therefore face "double stigma" (Kowalewski 1988: 211).[5] Stigma also may be more pronounced for PHAs who belong to other groups associated with social exclusion (e.g. PHAs of colour or the impoverished), who also may be discriminated against on the basis of membership in a non-hegemonic or relatively disenfranchised group. It may also vary during the course of the disease as the manner in which individuals personalize their illness, and the strategies they use to manage their social relationships, are linked to the progression of the disease in a process referred to by Alonzo and Reynolds (1995: 303) as the "stigma trajectory."

Furthermore, the stigma of AIDS may be extended to people of colour, IDUs (intravenous/injecting drug user), and gay people who are *not* infected with HIV (Kowalewski 1992). In other words, members of these groups who have not tested positive may be treated automatically as if they have, simply by virtue of shared membership in so-called 'risk groups'.[6] Similarly, through this process of symbolic contamination, AIDS stigma may even be extended to objects once owned or touched by PHAs, such as cars, hotel beds, sweaters, and drinking glasses. These objects are disdained because they remind people of the associated PHAs and so evoke negative thoughts and feelings similar to those that PHAs themselves evoke (Pryor and Reeder 1993).

In one US case in 1990, when an HIV-positive man's car slipped out of gear and rolled into a neighbour's fence, the neighbour was advised by police to wash with a disinfectant, as if contact with the car via contact with the damaged fence also constituted contact with the PHA (and as if casual contact with a PHA could lead to HIV transmission, and as if 'disinfectant' would make a difference). After news of the owner's seropositivity got around, 19 children were removed from the school where his children were enrolled (Pryor and Reeder 1993).

In addition to objects, then, stigma can contaminate people associated with PHAs even if they do not share risk-group membership. Goffman (1963) has called this type of stigma extension 'courtesy stigma'.[7] Carers and family members may suffer enormously as a result of this, experiencing loss of friends and harassment (Powell-Cope and Brown 1992) in addition to the eventual demise and loss of the PHA(s) with whom they are associated.

While gay, or drug-using, or minority PHAs may be stigmatized both as PHAs and as gays or IDUs or people of colour, the relationship between the multiple prejudices they face (prejudice related to AIDS *per se* and prejudice related to drug use or homosexuality or race) and the interchangeability of them is uncertain. Further, not all AIDS stigma is symbolic in nature. Crandall *et al.* (1997) have suggested that "the functional, illness aspects of HIV infection may be a primary source of AIDS-related stigmatization" (p. 103). They conducted studies about attitudes to a fictitious disease to see how people's attitudes changed according to the contagiousness, treatability and severity of the illness. When the fictitious disease was presented as relatively minor, temporary, treatable, or non-contagious, its stigma was reduced substantially.

Other studies have shown similar findings. For example, using data from a two-wave national telephone survey carried out with a national probability sample of US adults, Herek and Capitanio demonstrated that "intentions to avoid PWAs appeared to be shaped largely by concerns about HIV transmission" (1998: 22). While their subjects could easily be divided between people concerned primarily about what AIDS symbolizes and people concerned primarily about AIDS contagion, most individuals held both types of concerns simultaneously. Herek and Capitanio found that instrumental concerns (fear of contagion) explained the bulk of avoidance for both groups. Fear of contagion, rather than aversion to symbolic factors, is also identified in the literature as the prime concern of health care workers treating PHAs (see Chapter 8).

Notwithstanding that HIV infection may be deadly and, in a very restricted sense, is contagious, the threat of AIDS contagion has been exaggerated by many. Herek explains that hypervigilance, or unrealistic fears about one's risk for HIV infection, may come about when people lack a clear understanding of how HIV infection works. They may draw to mind what they know about other viral illnesses, such as colds or flu that may be transmitted by air or by touch. A prevalent

18

assumption in the 1980s was that mosquitoes could transmit AIDS, like malaria. Use of such easily available models of contagion can lead to miscalculations and over-estimations of personal risk (Herek 1990). But extreme fears of contagion may only exist in regard to transmission events over which one has little control or those which are highly unlikely (being bitten by a madman with AIDS, say, or contracting an infection when receiving treatment from an infected health care worker). People seem to be optimistically biased when it comes to real potential vectors, such as in their own sex lives (Sobo 1995b; Weinstein 1984, 1989).

Miscalculations of personal risk notwithstanding, concerns about transmission can be very real and are the basis of much AIDS stigma. The study referred to above by Crandall *et al.* (1997), however, demonstrated that without "a complete swamping of the field by the instrumental properties of the illness, the symbolic properties had a real impact" (p. 109). That is, when presented with alternate descriptions of two mildly ill men, one homosexual and the other not, and alternate descriptions of the fictitious disease said to have infected them, one linked with homosexuality and the other not, research subjects demonstrated more propensity toward social rejection in the homosexual or homosexuality-linked cases.

Most claims related to the symbolic role in the rejection of PHAs cite the association between homophobia and negative attitudes toward AIDS. In their work, Crandall *et al.* (1997) found that attitudes towards homosexuals correlated with a number of beliefs and attitudes, such as racism, rejection of fat people, and the belief that laziness leads people to become welfare recipients. This adds further complexity to the link between homophobia and rejection of PHAs as it suggests that high levels of homophobia are correlated with "a rejection of deviants of many sorts" (p. 110).[8] Thus, deviance in general may be more important than homosexuality *per se* in explaining the stigma of AIDS. Notwithstanding, homosexuality and AIDS are tightly linked in the public imagination – a point we return to below (regarding the complex links between homophobia and the rejection of PHAs, see also Abelove 1994; Herek 1997; Herek and Capitanio 1998; Pryor and Reeder 1993; Watney 1994).

Victim blaming

Stigma, inherently linked with deviance, has been shown in general to be greater where the stigmatized have a contagious disease that poses a danger or presents a peril to others (Jones *et al.* 1984; Alonzo and Reynolds 1995). It is also greater where the origin of a person's condition may be blamed on his or her own behaviour or thoughts (Crandall and Moriarty 1995; Jones *et al.* 1984; De Jong 1980). People with HIV who have been infected sexually or through sharing needles to inject drugs – both deviant behaviours that also can be seen as the personally controllable origin of infection – are thus particularly vulnerable to 'victim blaming'.

Gender expectations regarding power and autonomy also may come into play when evaluating the degree to which a person has control over whether they are infected or not. For example, Borchert and Rickabaugh (1995) found that, regardless of mode of infection, middle-class college undergraduates held women less responsible for their HIV infections than men: "Male targets were rated as exerting more control over HIV infection, regardless of the mode of transmission" (p. 664). While, as Borchert and Rickabaugh caution, "The schema of 'woman with AIDS' may be so underdeveloped that distinguishing and responding to female targets based on mode of HIV transmission is not likely" (p. 664), it seems that the lack of control generally attributed to women in contrast to men is what led to this finding.[9]

At an early stage in the AIDS pandemic, popular culture divided people with HIV into the 'innocent' (which included children, those infected through blood transmissions, etc.), and the 'guilty' (gay and bisexual men, drug users, and sex workers). Members of the former group were absolved from blame whereas members of the latter, deemed responsible for their own infection, were viewed as having got what they asked for. One-fifth of Herek's national US phone sample, polled in 1990–91, believed that "PWAs deserved their illness" (1997: 208), and a street survey conducted in 1993 by Green suggested that this viewpoint was shared by a minority of people in Scotland (Green 1995a; see Chapter 11).

The idea that PHAs 'get what they deserve' for engaging in risky behaviour "may represent a need to believe that the epidemic is controllable and that one can be safe by avoiding certain behaviors and following certain rules" (Herek 1990: 129). That is, it may be a coping strategy that helps people handle a horrible disease that has no cure. The threat of illness as a consequence of, or retribution for, socially deviant behaviour – a common concept cross-culturally, seen in relation to a multitude of ills – also serves to motivate people to follow social and cultural rules (Loustaunau and Sobo 1997; *cf.* McCrystal 1995).

This view is supported by some of those who fall ill. For example, Grove *et al.* (1997) found that middle-class US women with HIV and AIDS tended to "reproduce the dominant cultural representations of AIDS" (p. 335), drawing "on the cultural dichotomy between 'us' (nice girls) and 'them' (outsiders)" (p. 334) to "elicit sympathy without being marginalized" (p. 332). This strategy may help absolve themselves in their own and, they hope, in others' eyes, but by playing the 'innocent victim', they perpetuate the retributional model and support stigmatization of (other) PHAs.

The notion that PHAs are being punished for their past actions is supported by the modern Western[10] tendency to view individuals as, in many ways, masters of their own destinies. In this model, behaviour is voluntary; risk taking therefore is intentional and people who wilfully expose themselves to the possibility of infection have only themselves to blame. In the configuration of Western individualism generally assumed in relation to AIDS risk, there are no macro-level constraints on decisions; there is no coercion or involuntary risk taking. All action – even habitual action – is seen as the result of rational calculation that disclaims risk is a relative concept (Rhodes 1995). We discuss the shortcomings in accepted definitions of risk in Chapter 3; here, we are most interested in the construction of HIV infection as an outcome that individuals are personally responsible for.

While the proposition that infection with HIV is a personally controllable event is an important aspect of AIDS stigma in the USA and UK, reluctance to apply this proposition to oneself, as seen in what Sobo (1993a, 1995b) has termed 'Wisdom Narratives', 'Monogamy Narratives', and 'Betrayal Narratives', seems to run high. In the latter two story forms, one praises one's relationship choices, demonstrating that AIDS education messages are not personally relevant. In Betrayal Narratives, examples of which are found in Ward (1993b) and Grove *et al.* (1997), people disclaim personal responsibility for their infections; they blame betrayal for their infection with HIV. All three narrative forms reflect the same ambivalence about accepting responsibility for infection that fuels much of the rumour mongering and storytelling[11] that surrounds AIDS.

The socio-cultural functions of storytelling

MacIntyre (1985) explains that the human is a "story-telling animal" (p. 216), and that story telling is an integral part of making sense of society. We use stories in educating ourselves about cultural expectations and in generating action. Moreover, our reflection upon the stories that we find ourselves a part of is a crucial step in the process of identity construction and maintenance. In Monogamy and Wisdom Narratives, for example, people explain cultural ideals for relationships and make claims to have lived up to them. In Betrayal Narratives, they maintain their identities as 'good' people by laying the blame for infection on deceitful outside sources.

All of our stories or narratives, MacIntyre explains, have "some at least partly determinate conception of the final *telos*" (1995: 219). This *telos* (end; reason or goal) relates to some conception of morality. That is, all stories entail models of how the moral world should, ideally, be. So, by telling stories about AIDS and the people with it, we educate ourselves as to our culture's morals, norms and goals. And in most AIDS-related stories, the moral telos is demonstrated for a hypothetically seronegative audience. In stories about PHAs, the teller maintains personal distance from HIV, and the PHA serves as object, not subject.

The health protection scenario

One of the stories told about PHAs has to do with public health. We are not concerned (in this book) with the nature – or virtue – of official recommendations regarding serostatus information sharing, but self-disclosure of positive HIV serostatus to sexual partners is viewed by most as a mandatory health-protecting action. We call this view the 'Health Protection Scenario' (Sobo 1997). This scenario, in which certain actions are to be played out, entails several assumptions.

First, non-disclosure is bad and, by extension, non-disclosers are evil people. A second assumption is that self-disclosure will be accompanied by safer sex, if any (e.g. condom use). Self-disclosure talk does not always lead to safer sex action, as HIV-positive people know, and as some researchers (e.g. Green 1994a; Perry *et al.* 1990b, 1994) are starting to allow (and see Chapter 10).

Further, while some people see safer sex as good for HIV-positive people, in that it might protect against the intake of germs, the Health Protection Scenario gives highest priority to the health of the uninfected (seronegative). Those who already are seropositive tend not to figure in this scenario, except as potential infective agents.

That a supposedly objective public health message might comprise such moralizing commentary should not surprise us. Bailey has shown how morally persuasive rhetoric can underwrite policy decisions in even the most logic-oriented environments (e.g. 1983). Abelove (1994), Bolton (1992), Treichler (1992; 1993), Watney (1994), and many others have written extensively on the mainstream mores entailed in HIV education messages aimed at the non-positive population. For example, Abelove (1994) shows how the late 1980s repackaging of AIDS as a matter of concern for all people and not just gay men served to reinforce "regulative positions about sex and the family" (p. 4). This led safer sex messages to focus on "the usual hierarchy of sexual behaviors," which culminates in "penetrative-receptive procreative intercourse" (p. 13), while maintaining "silence on sexual options that may be subversive of the family" (p. 14). This also served to deflect attention away from the suffering of gay men, who as we write still comprise by far the largest portion of PHAs in Britain and the USA.

Waldby *et al.* (1995) examined representations of HIV and AIDS in medical textbooks and found similar normative biases. One textbook, for example, contrasts the bodies of gay men and IDUs with those of "normal" people (p. 23), reinforcing an essentialistic sense of difference. In medical writing, PHAs cannot "distinguish self from non-self" (p. 32); they have literally undergone "identity colonization" (p. 30) in the sense that their own genetic material has been colonized by HIV for use in its own reduplication. With changed DNA, PHAs are no longer the people they used to be. An alternative reading, and one that demands little understanding of genetics, is that the gay or drug using aspect of self is an enemy, as deserving of destruction as any harmful microbe.

The horror story

Similar biases are very clearly seen in non-disclosure rumours or horror stories that people recount to one another. In these stories, seronegative and seropositive people are explicitly contrasted along overtly moral lines. Serostatus *per se* is not the chief dimension of distinction here. As Watney (1994) and others have argued, AIDS is "a powerful condenser for a great range of social, sexual and psychic anxieties" (p. 9). Kane (1994) explains that through a "set of signifying practices" in which "risk behaviors qua groups" are conceptually isolated then united, AIDS – and so the groups associated with it – is transformed into "a mandala for public dread, a black hole for cast-off projections" (p. 3).

Watney (1994) points out that "AIDS has been mobilized to embody a variety of perceived threats to individual and social stability [and one of its principal uses has been] to stabilize the figure of the heterosexual family unit" (p. 10). Abelove (1994), Bolton (1992) and others have said the same. They argue that the horrifying (diseased, dying) figure of the PHA, which doubles for the figure of the cultural failure or fugitive, is used to frighten people into behaving according to the cultural expectation for 'clean and sober' heterosexual monogamy.

According to Watney (1994), this happens in two ways. Firstly, PHAs are publicly portrayed when at death's door; that is, the PHA's body is introduced under circumstances, or in a condition, in which any possibility of identification with – or desire for – that body is denied and difference is highlighted. We see the "dreaded object of desire [only] in the final moments of its own apparent self-destruction" (p. 53). Death is the price the PHA pays for contravening the laws of nature in comporting sexually with not women but men, or for injecting drugs, or engaging in prostitution, or all three. According to mainstream constructions, all of these bodies house evil deviance and evil bodies come to evil ends. There is nothing unique about this kind of thinking; health problems serving as punishments for social deviance are common across cultures and across times. The structural function of health-related anxiety is a common ethnographic theme (Loustaunau and Sobo 1997).

So: fear of a horrible death from AIDS, reinforced by the unimaginability of occupying the quintessential PHA's body, terrorizes people into self-regulated monogamous heterosexual family life – at least theoretically. People also are terrorized by the idea of meeting PHAs in their pre-cadaverous state; this is the second way that the figure of the PHA enforces social and cultural norms. "Instead of being regarded as threatened, people with AIDS become threatening," Watney says (1994: 24). The simple threat of being reminded of latent desires, or of ever-impending death, is compounded by the 'normal-looking' PHA. The threat aroused in the self-assumed seronegative individual by the asymptomatic PHA is that of deception: of not being able to discern what is real, what is good. And when one lives in a world of artifice and deceit, one solution is to reject illicit lifestyles and keep close to home, near to the family.

Urban legends

Popular AIDS tales reflect and help to maintain a widespread fear of being lied to or manipulated by unethical PHAs. Urban legends warning of beautiful HIV-positive charmers who enchant and then have unprotected sex with unsuspecting seronega-tive[12] people in order to spread the virus abound (cf. Farmer 1992; Turner 1993). Moreover, there have been a number of highly publicized cases in which HIV-positive individuals had unprotected sex with others while concealing their seropositivity.

Take, for example, the story of Gaetan Dugas or 'Patient Zero'. Bolton notes that after the 1987 publication of Shilts's *And the Band Played On*, which chronicled not only Dugas's progression from HIV infection to death but also his plenteous sexual liaisons, Dugas's story "was given extensive coverage and the role of his sexual escapades in spreading AIDS around the continent was highlighted" (Bolton 1992: 20). Dugas was vilified despite the fact that he could not have known as we do today the role of sexual intercourse in HIV transmission – and despite the essential part he played in helping epidemiologists to describe that role. Bolton, who also examines the case of HIV-positive prostitute Fabian Bridges, who allegedly inten-tionally infected his clients, points out, "In both of these cases the promiscuous individual was blamed for continuing to have sex knowingly and intentionally without concern for the consequences to his partners, thereby linking promiscuity with psychopathology (Bersani 1988) and sickness with crime (Quam 1990: 34)" (Bolton 1992: 20; citations in original).

Another highly publicized case with similar undertones occurred in 1995, in Ireland. After hearing the confession of a woman who had come asking forgiveness for purposefully infecting five men, a priest made it his duty to warn his parishioners. He spoke to them in church about, as one of Britain's broadsheets reported, "an HIV-infected 'Angel of Death' vengefully spreading the virus to men" (McCrystal 1995). The woman was an outsider, having moved to the parish after living in a big city.

The priest's announcement was said by one reporter (McCrystal 1995) to have "shocked his ... parishioners into sudden apocalyptic dread;" the "townspeople openly expressed communal penitence." One man pronounced, "We've gone too far down the promiscuous road." That such a thing could happen was taken as a warning meant to return the townsfolk to the righteous path. Stories of premarital sex and adultery were related to the reporting journalist. The specific alleged acts of non-disclosure were used as a springboard to a general discussion of a broad set of social, cultural, and moral expectations relating to family formation, rural-urban distinctions, and the related domain of regional politics.[13]

While non-disclosure may in many cases be motivated by loving intentions and a desire for intimacy (a motivation we return to in later chapters), the discourse of blame, deceit, and culpability is reflected in what we call the 'Myth of the Seropositive Monster' (Sobo 1997). This myth has many local forms but these tend to follow a general pattern (*cf.* Turner 1993). An 'innocent' person is seduced by and then intentionally infected by an evil AIDS 'carrier'.

For example, a friend of a friend's cousin meets a promising woman or man and the two go out on a date. The date goes very well. In fact, the evening becomes so romantic that the cousin is overcome by loving feelings and the couple ends up having sex. The next morning, the object of the cousin's affection has vanished. In his or her stead, in the bathroom, on the mirror, in red lipstick or maybe shaving foam, is a message stating that the cousin has been infected with HIV. The Myth of the Seropositive Monster may be modern in content but its form is very old. It follows a well-known narrative course: that of the beautiful temptress, enchantress, witch, or devil who seduces innocent youth away from the righteous road and onto the path of destruction.

In the Myth of the Seropositive Monster, the PHA serves as a prop in a lesson on how *not* to behave as a member of our community. Cross-culturally common 'us–them' thinking pervades AIDS rumours. But the apparently separate domains of insider and outsider, us and them, good and evil, the uninfected and the PHAs, are not actually separate after all when the PHA is asymptomatic, and that is what is frightening to the audience the story is intended for. Borders are permeable, crossed and penetrated, in very intimate ways (e.g. during penetrative sex, when people may be particularly emotionally and physiologically vulnerable to deception by a PHA).

Who is the subject?

Stories of non-disclosure are told as stories of concealment; self-disclosure is talked about as a thing that *did not happen*. Further, these stories are told from the sero-negative person's point of view; the seropositive person is discounted, being cast as criminal and incorrigible. This is the case even with the Betrayal Narrative, in which the speaker is cast as having been taken advantage of; the PHA is not a trustworthy entity. The Myth of the Seropositive Monster and the Health Protection Scenario go even further. Both give priority to the health of the seronegative. And both are morality tales in which the danger of non-prescriptive sex is death.[14]

In addition to being a lethal biological entity and a devastating physical disease, HIV is a socially and culturally significant illness state. It reflects or transmits to others the news that those infected with the virus are not acting as members of our group are meant to. They have broken too many social rules and therefore have been punished. And this – plus the threat of not noticing it, of being deceived by the PHA – is an important component of AIDS stigma. The content of AIDS-related stories such as those we have just examined demonstrate that the fear of being duped, being lied to, being taken advantage of, and not being in control combine with homophobia and fear of catching AIDS to form a primary root of AIDS stigma.

Story, identity, social risk and reality

The AIDS narratives we have reviewed are not only used as warnings to damper deviance. They also are used by PHAs as they rethink and redefine who they are and where they are going. In this book, we investigate the degree to which AIDS's social risk affects the HIV-positive person's perceived quality of life and his or her negotiation of social relationships. We contend that this depends to some degree on the ways in which AIDS-related riskiness – here, the stigmatized identity component related to AIDS – is incorporated into the PHAs vision of who s/he now is. It also depends on how others view or act toward PHAs.

AIDS stigma in action

Hostile attitudes and discrimination

AIDS stigma is complex and multi-faceted. Both symbolic and instrumental in nature, it includes beliefs that PHAs are: intrinsically different from others; responsible for their condition; and should have their behaviour restricted so that they do not threaten others with HIV transmission (Green 1995a), even if accidentally. In any given social situation, some or all of these aspects of AIDS stigma can emerge to taint interaction.

One does not have to look far for examples of outright discrimination against people with HIV: many countries deny PHAs entry, insurance companies deny life insurance, and people with HIV (e.g. in the USA and Cyprus[15]) have been convicted for 'knowingly' infecting another person. PHAs, and even people merely perceived to be HIV-positive, "have been fired from their jobs, driven from their homes, and socially isolated" (Herek and Glunt 1993: 231). Research in the late 1980s showed that "a significant minority of the American public consistently endorsed repressive measures" including mandatory testing and branding the infected with tattoos (Herek 1997: 194). While PHA quarantine laws have never been passed in the USA, just over one-third (35.5%) of Herek's 1990–91 national phone sample supported quarantine and just under one-third (29.1%) favoured the public release of names of PHAs (p. 208).

Whilst in Britain it has been shown that a majority of people support the rights of PHAs (Brook 1988; Wellings and Wadsworth 1990), a telephone survey of 25,000 people in Glasgow, Edinburgh and London identified a small minority of males over 40 as having extreme punitive attitudes towards people with AIDS (Nisbet and McQueen 1993). Research has confirmed that in other parts of Europe, too, a minority of people hold highly restrictive and repressive attitudes towards people with HIV (Ralston et al. 1992; Elliott et al. 1992; Dab et al. 1989). Such opinions tend to be fairly consistently patterned according to social characteristics. Being older, non-white, less well educated, and politically 'to the right' is related to prejudiced attitudes (Peruga and Calentano 1993).

It should, however, be noted that a survey carried out by the Health Education Authority in Britain in 1989 and again in 1996 found that attitudes were becoming more tolerant (National AIDS Trust and Health Education Authority 1997). The same may be occurring in the USA. Notwithstanding a possible liberalization of societal attitudes, a recent review of the literature concludes, "It is clear that fears, misconceptions and negative attitudes to individuals with AIDS remain common among the general public" (Välimäki et al. 1998: 757). It also is clear that many people with HIV in Britain and USA still suffer discrimination and AIDS remains a highly stigmatized condition.

Impact on social support

There is concern that AIDS stigma may lead to the diminution of PHAs' support networks. This shrinkage may in turn have adverse affects upon their psychological and physical well being. This process which may result in social isolation is thought to be one of the most debilitating aspects of chronic illness (Royer 1998). Despite common assumptions that social networks get smaller following diagnosis there is little clear evidence of this (we present our own data in Chapter 11). There may, however, be subtle changes in social relationships in response to an HIV diagnosis, such as close friendships becoming closer whereas casual friends become less valued (Hays *et al.* 1990).

The majority of studies on social support and HIV to date have focused upon gay white males in the USA (see the review by Green 1993), who are reported to have better support than those belonging to other transmission groups (e.g. Eich *et al.* 1990).[16] These findings may not be generalizable to all or other people with HIV. Social support structures and social networks vary according to social, economic and cultural factors (differences that are discussed in Chapter 11).

Notwithstanding variation between PHAs, all face potentially negative social experiences when their stigma is disclosed. In-depth studies of people with HIV report that public stigmatization may threaten identity (Sandstrom 1990), lead to loss of self-esteem (Siegel and Krauss 1991; Bennett 1990), and have a greater impact than the physical disorder (King 1989; Crowther 1992). Whilst there is plenty of evidence that people with HIV are stigmatized, the processes through which stigmatization operates, and the degree to which felt and enacted stigma are matched, are not well-understood. Our own work suggests that felt stigma among PHAs is very high. The impact of felt stigma may lead PHAs to overestimate discrimination and other negative reactions, and it may lead to a level of concealment and a fragmentation of identity that is itself damaging. Before we examine the validity of these hypotheses, we must explain just what we mean by social risk. We do so in the next chapter.

Notes

1 Portions of this chapter are based, with kind permission, on an analysis that Sobo published previously (1997).

2 There does exist a popular (i.e. non-academic) qualitative experience-oriented literature but, for the most part, academics do not cite it. This is ostensibly due to credibility concerns. The writings are deemed too unscholarly (e.g. including no citations) or too political (e.g. having fully articulated action agendas).

3 The amount of research focused specifically on self-disclosure (as opposed to disclosure made by a third party) is growing but still not large. A review of it is included in Chapter 9. While a few scholars have investigated intentions to self-disclose (e.g. Kegeles et al. 1988), or looked at the costs and benefits of disclosure (e.g. Holt et al. 1998), and some individual case studies of non-disclosure have been documented (e.g. Chiodo and Tolle 1992), much of the available literature, limited as it is, takes the form of guidelines for HIV/AIDS counsellors (e.g. Green 1989a; Sherr 1991). The advice offered is generally impressionistic and suggestive, and although it may be useful to counsellors, it is not research based (much of that which is based on research is undertaken in regard to chronic diseases or conditions other than AIDS).

4 This attribution pattern was no doubt based on actual historical and contemporary experience of such prejudice.

5 In places like Africa, however, where homosexual transmission is much less frequent and most of those infected are heterosexual women, the association between HIV and homosexuals may be much less intense (Pryor and Reeder 1993: 271–272).

6 Regarding problems inherent in the 'risk group' concept, see Glick-Schiller (1992).

7 The logic that underlies both types of associative stigma is the logic of contagion – a logic shown by Frazer (1979) to exist cross culturally (see also Rozin and Nemeroff 1990).

8 This links in with Conserve's (1964) concept of centrality of belief systems. Although his focus is upon political attitudes, the notion that there are clusters of ideas around a topic and that these are particularly tightly held together if the topic concerns attitudes towards a particular social group, is relevant here.

9 Notwithstanding, women were more likely to be held accountable for their drug addictions than men were. This was probably due to assumptions regarding their violation of female role expectations in taking up drug injection – role expectations that, at the same time, posit women as sexually docile rather than as instigators in the sexual arena (see also Grove et al. 1997; Lawless et al. 1996; Sacks 1996).

10 While we are aware of the debate that surrounds the use of the term 'Western' we have elected to use it in the lay sense (i.e. in reference to the hegemonic post-industrial, post-colonial Judeo-Christian late capitalist culture shared by wealthy Northern nations such as the USA, Scotland, and England) because that debate is beyond the scope of this project.

11 We use the term 'stories' in the broadest sense, to encompass what might otherwise be termed 'rumours' or 'urban legends' or even 'discourses' or 'scenarios' (as in the "health

protection scenario" to be described in the next section), as well as tales that follow the narrative forms just outlined.

12 Many people assumed to be seronegative actually have not been tested. This fact should be borne in mind as the reader considers sex between a PHA and any other individual who has not explicitly tested positive for HIV antibodies.

13 The woman had recently moved to the parish after having lived in London, which has important implications in relation to the Irish-English argument.

14 The shortcomings of education messages promoting prescriptive sex (e.g. that between long-term partners or spouses) as protective are examined elsewhere by Sobo (1993a, 1995b).

15 There was much news coverage in the UK about the arrest of Pavlos Georgiou, the Cypriot partner of a British woman Janette Pink. Mrs Pink accused her lover of having a relationship with her without disclosing his HIV-positive status and subsequently infecting her with HIV. He was found guilty but not imprisoned.

16 This may only be so for men who identify as gay and are self-proclaimed members of a 'gay community'. Rural or closeted homosexual men may not find themselves socially supported.

Chapter 3

The landscape of risk: danger, identity, and HIV

Living in a 'Risk Society'

Whilst many disagree about the factors that produce a 'risk society' (Beck 1992), it is undeniable that there is increased awareness of danger in people's everyday lives. A scientific-like consciousness of risk informs many everyday assessments and decisions (Ericson and Haggerty 1997). As Giddens puts it, "Awareness of risks seeps into the actions of almost everyone" (1991: 111).

A glance through any newspaper (in this example the little known *Clacton and Harwich Evening Gazette,* UK) illustrates the pervasiveness of risk in our lives. Stories in just one issue (8 July 98) alert us to the many dangers threatening local society such as: a 12-year-old stealing a pensioner's bag, a man being knocked off his bicycle; theft of diverse possessions ranging from cars to a centenarian tortoise; rain threatening strawberry crops; and telephone kiosks being vandalized. Other stories focus specifically upon the management of risk to avoid such pitfalls. Health chiefs are criticized for the death of a prisoner killed by his schizophrenic cellmate. Angry residents call for the relocation of a bus shelter due to fears that in its present site "it is dangerous and an accident waiting to happen" (p. 6).

Risk is also salient in national news stories. On the radio news this morning in England we heard that the British Medical Association are debating action to address the problem that one in ten hospital patients leave with an infection caught on the

31

wards. There were also reports that women with silicone implants are suing the manufacturers on the grounds that the implants made them sick.

An increased awareness of possible risks is not confined to the UK but is common throughout the Western world. In the USA today, CNN's national evening news show reported stories of people dying from medical 'mistakes' and being given prescriptions for the 'wrong' medications. A health maintenance organization (HMO) magazine received in the morning mail contained, among other warning essays, a story on food-borne illness called 'The E. Coli Question' and, on the same page, 'Careful When Climbing', which informs us that "more than 30,000 people fall off ladders every year" *(Health-Net Bulletin* 1998: 6). The plastic bag that the bulletin arrived in was identified as a suffocation hazard for small children.

Risk appraisal and management are now key organizing principles in many institutions. There exists what Gabe (1995: 1) refers to as a "risk industry" which is institutionalized in societies and journals. Yet, there are few agreed definitions of the term 'risk,' often used interchangeably with 'danger' and 'hazard'. Further, risk research in different disciplines has been compartmentalized, resulting in fragmenta-tion, leading to what Hood and Jones (1996) call the "risk archipelago" rather than the risk literature. We seek in this section to clarify risk's definition and to discuss the shortcomings of certain conceptions of the term in relation to the central questions of this book.

The emergence of risk

The 'risk society', as conceptualized by Beck (1992), is a paradox of late modernity, in which progress and industrialization have arrived hand in hand with environmental hazards that threaten the ecosystem and the health of humanity.[1] Awareness of environmental and industrial hazards conceived in terms of calculable risk has facilitated an awareness of internal or lifestyle risks over which we ostensibly have some control.[2] What a person eats, drinks or smokes, what job one does, what hobbies one has, who one sleeps with (and how) are all part of a health-risk profile, which posits a person as more or less vulnerable to a host of illnesses, disabilities and diseases.

Although the equation between lifestyle and health status has been in existence since the first societies began, and is seen cross-culturally in the form of illness explanations (e.g. Sobo 1993b), the AIDS pandemic brought the specific concept of 'lifestyle risk' into sharp focus. The term 'risk behaviour' and the concepts of 'risk groups' and 'risk reduction' came into common parlance following the advent of AIDS. These epidemiological categories, by which behaviour is reduced to easily measurable, decontextualized units, were accepted by social researchers, largely without question (Rhodes 1995), in part due to the cultural hegemony of the industrial-scientific mode of thought (Adam 1998). Our reliance on these terms and the categories they represent has led to a plethora of studies about risky sexual behaviour. The notion that gay men and drug users are both 'high risk' groups in terms of AIDS is widely held in the USA and UK; and health promotion to reduce transmission focuses on 'risk reduction' messages, such as use of clean needles or condoms.

This asocial mode of understanding risk and assessing it has its roots, for socio-cultural reasons introduced shortly, in mathematical calculations of probability. Probability *per se* is a relatively neutral concept: something will or will not happen and that is that. But in modern parlance, risk is used to signify danger or hazards. Further, risk assessment is part of an approach that sees unfortunate events as both predictable and avoidable (Lupton 1995). According to Beck, "Basically, one is no longer concerned with obtaining something 'good', but rather with preventing the worst" (Beck 1992: 49).

Still, risk behaviour does have potential benefits. Risk, notes Bauman (1992), belongs to the discourse of gambling, and people gamble in order to win. This is important in the context of a study about social risk: taking risks may sometimes have negative outcomes such as rejection, isolation or loss of status; at other times, taking risks may have positive results such as increased support, love and close-ness.[3] Further, for some, the immediate excitement or heightened arousal entailed in taking a risk makes risk-taking its own reward.

Systems of assessing and managing risk

Adam argues that industrialization encouraged "industrial habits of mind" (1998: 58) – ways of seeing and thinking about the world that favoured quantification, calculation, and compartmentalization. The mathematical theory of probability has been used to produce models of risk and risk management for use in industry (see Dickson 1991) where, Adam argues, expectations of certainty and predictability reign. Mathematical tools, however, are clearly limited when it comes to interpreting social behaviour, and their use by epidemiologists to measure and quantify health risks is problematic in this light (Frankenberg 1994; Peterson and Lupton 1996). Indeed, many would argue that any objective quantification of risk to explain human behaviour is inherently flawed as "both the adverse nature of particular events and their probability are inherently subjective" (Adams 1995: 9; see also Frankenberg 1994).

Adams's comment on adversity needs little elaboration: losing one's left hand at the wrist is certainly more adverse for the concert pianist than the news anchor person. The subjectivity of risk calculation, which is a bit more complex, is well illustrated by Kaufert and O'Neil's (1993) examination of the diverse discourses and concepts of risks in childbirth used by physicians and Inuit women living in a remote area of the Canadian Arctic. The physicians combined the epidemiological language of risk, derived from statistics, with cases of actual or near disaster that they had witnessed or heard about. Such 'facts' were set within a context of vulnerability and responsibility that led them to perceive childbirth as an inherently dangerous process. But the Inuit women's language of risk was set within the context of the "general 'riskiness' of human existence (including assumptions about risk in childbirth) [that] were linked with the physical environment in which they lived and with their recent history and cultural traditions" (p. 48). As a result, they viewed childbirth as an essentially safe, natural process. The degree to which a behaviour is culturally 'normal' seems to affect one's subjective view of it as risky or not (Rhodes 1995).

Differences between lay and 'expert' perceptions of risk are also reported by Davison *et al.* (1991) with regard to lay beliefs about the risk of coronary heart disease, and in Roberts *et al.* (1992) study of childhood accidents in Glasgow, Scotland. Studies such as these highlight the difference between knowledge that is subjective and experientially based and that which is objective and based on science. The clarity of the line between these two types of knowledge has, however, been questioned by, among others, Carter (1995), Toft (1996) and Petersen and Lupton (1996), who argue that the assumption that risks, even those calculated on the basis of 'scientific knowledge', can be objectively defined and measured is erroneous. All risks and measurement of them are to a large extent subjective; the scientific 'facts' upon which many measures are based are themselves largely culturally constructed and subjective. Thus the two ways of conceptualizing risk proposed by Gifford (1986) – the 'scientific' approach and through lived experience – may not be mutually exclusive. This does not, of course, detract from the very powerful cultural position enjoyed by science, the mere reference to which ('science has proven' or 'scientists say') can clinch an argument, or at least silence one's opponent.

Notwithstanding the power of science, problems of relativity confront those who seek to pin down risk with objective numbers, and a cost-benefit approach to human behaviour is clearly limited (Carter 1996). Adam argues that a notion of risk based on assumptions of the possibility of calculation and control must fail when "causes and symptoms are separated by an open, unspecifiable time gap of invisible impact" (1998: 82), as they are in the case of acid rain, global warming, and HIV infection.

But it is not just a time gap that makes the possibility of calculation tenuous. The complexity of a given situation can make calculation a ridiculous exercise. Hart *et al.* (1992) clearly demonstrate that 'rational choice' models are not appropriate to explain risk behaviour within the complexities of everyday gay culture. The major shortcoming of socio-psychological models which attempt to construct risk as a single measurable object has to do with the fact that, in reality, many factors (social, political, cultural, etc.) may be involved. Further, as risk is socially organized in so many ways, taking the individual as the sole unit of analysis is a misguided methodological decision. Rhodes (1995) shows that risk calculation may be made on the social and not individual level: risk-related perceptions and actions often are socially organized or culturally determined and in this sense we contend that they may be understood as pre-rational givens.

A construction of risk that implies that all individuals are autonomous, equally powerful, and driven only by rational calculation is indefensible for other reasons as well. For example, processes deemed mundane or normal are not likely to lead to conscious considerations of risk at all, in part because they do not represent departures from the norm (Bloor 1995b). And any calculations that may in fact be made regarding habitual, everyday behaviours are more likely to be framed in terms of benefits than costs (Rhodes 1995).

Further, as Bloor's (1995a) study of male prostitutes' risk behaviour shows, perception of risk and rational calculating do not necessarily predict behaviour as we are sometimes constrained from acting according to rational decisions. This is often the case in social or sexual encounters as more than one person is involved and factors such as power and self-esteem come into play. Risk interaction frequently takes place on terms of gross inequality and just as one would expect a cyclist to fare worse than a lorry in a collision between the two, so one might expect an inexperienced young prostitute to derive different benefits from a sexual encounter than the more affluent and more powerful client.

Such shortcomings in risk theory are partially addressed by approaches that emphasize the 'situated rationality' of risk behaviour. These studies show how seemingly 'irrational' behaviour may be the logical outcome of a number of contradictory social pressures. This is well illustrated by Parson's (1992) study of the reproductive behaviour of women at risk of bearing children with the genetic disorder of Duchenne Muscular Dystrophy. Clinically irrational decisions against abortion were understandable in terms of the high value the deciding mothers placed on family formation, or their positive memories of a sibling with the disorder. Grinyer's work with midwives (1995) is similarly illustrative: midwives may increase their health risks by not wearing goggles and masks, but they decrease the social risk of damaging their relationship with the patient by avoiding the distancing use of protective gear.

But rationality is not situated in just one context, and the process of balancing or juggling risks in different domains of one's life is central to the interpretation of risk management we would like to present. Bloor (1995b) notes that many data used to support the situated rationality approach come from retrospective interview studies rather than studies done in natural settings, and therefore the validity of the narratives in terms of study goals is suspect. As Bloor (1995b) suggests, retrospective accounts may be presented as situated rationality but may have become so only in the telling (see also MacIntyre 1985).

Clearly the distinction between perceived and objective risks is not clear-cut. Even so-called 'objective' risks have a large judgmental component; values shape facts and facts shape values and neither can be separated (Fischhoff *et al.* 1984). Qualitative subjective judgements play an important part in both the assessment and management of risk, and such judgements are linked to cultural and social factors (Douglas and Wildavsky 1982; Douglas 1986, 1992). Accordingly, in this book we view risk as a social construct (and not as an objective measure), and we interpret PHAs' narratives of social risk behaviour from this perspective.

As Adam notes, "the language of risk assessment and calculation becomes inappropriate in process-phenomena that are time-space distantiated, contingent, [and] interconnected" (1998: 82). Notwithstanding, we seek not to replace that language but rather to draw attention to some of the understandings that it can carry when used casually or without contemplation. Because risk terminology is so prevalent in the AIDS literature, and in the discourse of our participants, rather than to try to replace it, we simply have sought to arrive at a more helpful definition of the term 'risk'. Otherwise, and as previous researchers (e.g. Hart and Boulton 1995) have argued, what people do when they assess their so-called risks will, by definition, be left out of the scholarly purview.

It is not just scholars who lack insight into their own problematic assumptions regarding the nature of risk. Our participants often exhibited the same "industrial habits of mind" (Adam 1998: 58) as those that lead scholars – including experts on AIDS – to the limited conceptualization of risk that we have been critiquing. Participants often appealed to the same taken-for-granted models in their interviews, for example in presenting to us lists of costs and benefits, and discussing decisions as if wholly rationally calculated. Further, as much public health discourse on AIDS is permeated with industrial risk rhetoric, the experience of the PHA is biased from the start toward perceiving all AIDS-related decisions in terms of weighing risk costs and benefits. The interpretation of the participants' testimonies presented in later chapters provides insight into the risk-related experiences that available models were inadequate for describing.

Risk and identity

To understand the process of personal (as opposed to industrial) risk assessment, we must take account of "people's social circumstances or own understandings of danger" (Carter 1996: 220). We argue that these are subtly bound up with their identities. From this perspective, Holland *et al.* (1990) describe the identity issues for a young woman trying to protect her sexual health who risks losing her reputation if she carries condoms, or her boyfriend if she insists on safer sex. Similarly, Sobo (1993a, 1995b) shows how even acknowledging risk for HIV infection from a partner (which HIV-protective condom use depends upon) may be too difficult and too dangerous for women whose identities hinge on their fulfilling cultural expectations regarding their relationships with men. So long as condom use suggests that partners are unfaithful and uncaring, many women will have nothing of it. For doing so would entail refiguring one's identity (see also Ratliff 1999).

The links between risk and identity are fundamental to an understanding of risk behaviour and each individual's risk behaviour has to be set within the context of the constraints, restrictions and priorities related to who s/he is. For example, the rock climber must expose him- or herself to a certain amount of danger on the rock face if s/he is to succeed in laying claim to that identity. Writes Carter (1996: 242):

> If the analysis of risk behaviour is to move forward, it must examine the articulation of risk with identity: the ways in which people use risk (either by avoidance or acceptance) reflexively to establish a sense of the self; the ways in which risk can be either a source of fear or pleasure; the risks that are imposed on some individuals because of their gender, sexual orientation, class, ethnicity, or desiring preferences; and the ways in which uncertainty and loss are given cultural meaning. The ways in which we all deal with danger and uncertainty are part of our identity, not separate from it.

Identity is thus an integral part of our perception and management of risk, both in terms of identities that entail and are supported by certain kinds of risk-taking, and in terms of risks that threaten certain identities and so must be avoided.

Moreover, and as the quote from Carter (1996: 242) suggests, particular identities – especially ethno-racial, gender, income or class identities – can and do entail risks that are structurally imposed. In this book we lack space to fully articulate a political economy perspective, but Singer (1998) has amply demonstrated how the structure of social relations that grows out of the modern system of economic production limits life options for select groups of people. People are exposed to or are expected to endure certain risks as a result of their position in this structure. The pattern of HIV's inter- and intra-national spread provides clear evidence for this, and we ask our readers to bear in mind the impact of structural forces when evaluating diverse participants' reported experiences.

Risk margins are thus structurally and culturally organized. The social organization of risk is seen not only in the differing risk margins of people of different statuses. It also is seen in the fact that our own risk limits rarely encompass cultural acts that we have been socialized to consider as mundane or everyday (Rhodes 1995) – until a change in circumstances makes even these practices seem dangerous.

Personal risk perimeters are constructed and maintained in relation to imagined others with whom we identify (healthy selves) and they separate us from those we would distance ourselves from (unhealthy others). The conceptual boundary between safety and danger is permeable, and "part of the danger that the 'other' represents is the threat (even if it is imaginary) that it may colonise the self rather than vice-a-versa" (Carter 1995: 143). The 'them' and 'us' mentality, which underpins stigma, thus also is salient in the process of risk assessment and management when identity's role in this process is taken into account. The notion of boundaries delineating 'safety' and 'danger' or 'self' and 'other' is employed by Bauman (1991) who refers to the "slimy," who threatens boundaries vital to native identity. The slimy is like a weed in a landscaped garden: an ambivalent entity that reaffirms randomness and demonstrates the limits of our control. The slimy is ambivalent (slippery) because it is not wholly 'other'; the weed is still a plant, and danger is not simply something outside of the garden wall. The slimy is a stranger who brings the outside inside and poisons "the comfort of order with suspicion of chaos" (Bauman 1991: 56).

The presence of the slimy is implicated in the institution of stigma, which Bauman sees as "a convenient weapon against the unwelcome ambiguity of the stranger. The essence of stigma is to emphasise the difference" (1991: 67). People who carry a stigma are thus the embodiment of the ambivalent dangerous 'other'. This challenges their identities and so their danger boundaries, which may be redrawn. For example, in the case of AIDS, social risks that were at one time well worth taking (e.g. sharing home truths to cement a relationship) or minimal (e.g. reviewing health history with the company doctor) may become too risky for consideration.

In AIDS symbolism, "The subordinate or marginalized other is culturally situated both as a physical danger to the healthy individual and as a symbolic danger to the social self. Disease in the already stigmatized other is the embodiment of moral pollution" (Crawford 1994: 1359). Rather than accept this otherness, however, PHAs may try to disassociate themselves from it and reaffirm their healthiness and thus their social centrality or 'us-ness'. Crossley shows how long-term HIV-positive individuals who describe themselves as 'healthy survivors' create "their own conceptions of 'self' and 'other' which microcosmically mirror typical processes of identity construction" (1997: 1863). This process has also been noted among other groups of people with chronic illness. Herzlich and Pierret describe how the phrase "I am not a sick person" was frequently voiced (1987: 224) in interviews with chronically ill people in France, and Kagawa-Singer (1993) noted that people with cancer in California generally described their health as 'good' or 'very good'. We revisit the links between AIDS and chronic illness in more depth in Chapter 5.

Landscapes of risk

Our notion of social risk is based upon the premise that risk is inextricably bound up with identity (Carter 1996), and our interpretation of PHAs' risk assessment and management is firmly situated in the nexus of this linkage. As identity is situational and multidimensional, so too is risk. Thus, like everyone else, PHAs must navigate and manage social risk within the 'landscape of risk' described by Davison (1991):

Everyone lives in a complex landscape of relative risk. Everyone ... [has] their own unique, personal landscape of risk – you can't quantify the landscape, as it is in a constant state of flux. What we fear changes with age, personal experience and with news from the outside world, and of course all of the elements are shot through with the random effects of fate and chance, the hand of God and notions of destiny. Our fluid, ever-changing landscapes of risk make it difficult to accept inflexible health education messages. We are led to both believe and disbelieve at the same time.

The 'landscape of risk' is fancifully illustrated by Adams (1995: 34) in a unique diagrammatic representation of what he calls "the dance of the risk thermostats." In this unusual diagram, 'risk thermostats' (models of a theory of risk-taking) of various sizes dance around each other whilst above them lightning strikes and an angel hovers to symbolize the natural and supernatural forces that overhang the dance floor.

The concept of a loose, ever-changing and moving landscape of risk stands in opposition to many of the more well-established (cost-benefit, rational action) ways of understanding risk in behavioural contexts (see Bloor 1995a; Gabe 1995; Carter 1996). Yet given the constantly changing landscape of risk, attempts at measuring, objectifying or even balancing risks are at best limited for, as Adams (1995: 29) notes:

> Risk is constantly in motion and it moves in response to attempts to measure it. The problems of measuring risk are akin to those of physical measurement in a world where everything is moving at the speed of light, where the act of measurement alters that which is being measured, and where there are as many frames of reference as there are observers.

In such a scenario, judging social and physical risk is a dynamic process as that which one seeks to judge is constantly changing.

As we soon show, each PHA navigates his or her own landscape of risk, which changes according to time and place. In light of the constant and dynamic change and flux ongoing in the risk landscape, we use the image of juggling to portray the process of risk management in everyday life. Each PHA, embodying the stigmatized unhealthy other, is involved in an improvised ballet, juggling balls of unequal weights and dimensions under conditions of shifting gravity on a moving floor. The act is not optional; it is an essential and ongoing effort to preserve a sense of selfhood. Keeping all the balls from falling requires constant surveillance and energy. Safety and danger are ambivalent constructions like Bauman's slippery weed (1991); a gesture of love may become the transmission route of a fatal illness and an encounter anticipated with fright may end happily after all.

What is social risk?

Risk in general is defined as the chance one takes that a given action will lead to a significant change. We have shown how risk management and perception is socio-culturally conditioned. A specifically social risk is a risk that, in addition to being socio-culturally conditioned, might alter one's social relations.

Social risk-taking, then, involves taking an action, engaging in a behaviour, or adopting an identity or an identity component that might alter one's social relations and so one's place in one's various social networks (e.g. familial, sexual, income-related, etc.) and one's position in society as a whole. For example, a person who pierces his or her lip might lose a job, alienate non-like-minded peers, get evicted – or gain a new peer group and impress the landlord and the boss.

Piercing or other body modifications are generally social risks for people living within, and desiring the esteem of, the dominant society in the USA or UK. But for others, body modifications are required for earning respect. The difference noted can be envisioned as a difference in the landscape of risk. Each individual occupies and must negotiate a landscape of risk that is in some senses generic, as many social risks are the same for all people across the board. However, in some senses, the landscape of risk is extremely individual, as individual circumstances, preferences, and goals as well as local mores affect the shape one's landscape takes.

People differ, their goals differ, their social networks differ, and so the landscapes of risk they have to negotiate also differ. Landscapes also change over time; they are not static, but grow and evolve with the individual. What was horrifyingly risky socially to the young adolescent in school can shrink vastly in significance in the eyes of a well-adjusted adult.

The especially risky risk landscape of the PHA

The landscape of risk alters immensely upon testing positive for HIV. Social risk increases tremendously in many cases as associating oneself with, or being otherwise associated with, this disease generally jeopardizes many of one's social relations. In this sense, being infected with HIV is a socially risky endeavour; PHAs are at increased social risk. Because of the stigma associated with AIDS, managing the social risk of an HIV identity is akin to juggling a grand piano, an anvil and a feather on a storm-tossed boat in a turbulent sea. One does well simply to stay afloat.

The possible erosion of social support for people with HIV and their potential isolation and loss of status due to the stigmatizing nature of the condition are cause for concern. When HIV infects members of already-marginalized groups, the stigma attached to it is layered upon pre-existing stigmata related to homophobia, negative feelings towards drug users (Herek and Glunt 1988), and deviance in general (Crandall *et al.* 1997). AIDS-related social risk-taking can, of course, lead to changes for the better. For example, while non-disclosure may enable one to continue to live an illness- and stigma-free life, at least until the onset of symptoms, disclosure may reveal formerly unrecognized support or lead to closer relationships with former contacts. But we are mostly concerned here with possible negative outcomes.

Dangers of disclosure

Much of the research on non-disclosure focuses on the experiences of men who have sex with men. Research carried out with mostly white, mostly educated, mostly well-off homosexual San Francisco men included an open-ended question regarding the decision to keep one's seropositivity secret (Hays *et al.* 1993). The study concerned disclosure to parents, friends, co-workers, clinicians, landlords and others as well as to primary partners. Many of the men decided not to disclose to certain people because they saw no benefit in doing so or because they felt that the costs would outweigh the benefits. Potential interpersonal costs included losing or damaging a relationship, causing another person undue stress, and having to deal with that person's emotional reactions to the news. The men also expressed concerns over revealing homosexuality and the possibility of the disclosee's verbal indiscretion (see also Siegel and Krauss 1991).

Desires for intimacy, continued social support, and smooth relations seem to play a large part in non-disclosure. So may a desire for physical safety: HIV-positive people have been shot or otherwise injured by partners after self-disclosing (*Baltimore Sun* 1993). Abandonment by an individual disclosed to also can threaten the self-discloser's physical well being, as when s/he has been living with or supported by that person. Moreover, self-disclosure can lead to job termination, housing discrimination, travel restrictions, denial of insurance and other practical problems. Discrimination such as this is widely reported in the media and through the gossip grapevines formed by social networks. It also is documented in the scientific literature (e.g. de Puy, Green, Molyneux, Roth, Schizas, Wilson, all in Fitzsimons *et al.* 1995; Ross and Hunter 1991; Alonzo and Reynolds 1995; Crandall and Coleman 1992).

PHAs seeking to avoid disclosure and resulting confrontations with stigma may create social distance or keep (or make) relationships and conversations superficial in order to avoid having to disclose serostatus (Herek 1990). They may "carefully structure social situations to minimize the risk of exposure" of their condition (p. 135). Signs of illness related to HIV may be cast as signs of less stigmatized diseases.

These and similar coping strategies do have certain benefits, but sometimes they backfire: one woman known to us (not a participant in this research) told her employer that she had lupus, a chronic degenerative disease. He immediately tried to engage her in an in-depth conversation about the disease – which his wife also suffered from. The woman, ill prepared to enter any dialogue regarding lupus, which she really knew very little about, had inadvertently placed herself in an awkward position indeed (see also Grove *et al.* 1997).

While this kind of outcome may be rare, such concealment-related coping strategies also can backfire in a more concrete sense, entailing dire costs in terms of health and well-being. PHAs may cut themselves off from potential sources of support at times when they would most benefit from it. They may "experience a great discrepancy between their public and private identities" (Herek 1990: 135), which can be disorienting. They may feel "they are living on a leash because they must stay close to home" where they can rest, reapply makeup (which might be used, for example, to cover lesions or fatigue), and otherwise refresh their "disguise" (p. 135). Maintenance of secrecy may be very stressful, and may heighten a person's sense of shame and contamination. Indeed, research among PHAs shows that those who feel stigmatized are also most likely to feel anxious, depressed or alienated from others and experience disruptions in normal social relationships (Crandall and Coleman 1992; Holt et al. 1998).

Disclosure may be as stressful as non-disclosure. Holt et al. (1998) report from their interviews with gay and bisexual men in the North of England that "disclosing one's HIV-status was an acute and recurrent stressor" (p. 49), even though it was also a mechanism for coping with the condition.

Studies of HIV-positive people's fears of disclosure are not numerous (for exceptions, see Holt et al. 1998; Hays 1993; Mason et al. 1995; Wolitski et al. 1998). But Mansergh et al. (1995) found that of the 684 HIV-positive men who took part in their study, those who had disclosed reported more favourable reactions from significant others than the non-disclosers in the study anticipated. And a study of the stigma associated with breast cancer found that family and friends of women being treated did not withdraw physically or psychologically; on the contrary, they provided increased emotional support (Bloom and Kessler 1994). So stigma does not necessarily diminish emotional support from close social contacts.

Notwithstanding, AIDS is a comparatively new illness and one that affects mainly relatively young people. In most locations in the UK and USA, people have little experience dealing with young people with any chronic illness; in some areas, few people have had experience dealing with people of any age with AIDS. Social contacts to whom PHAs disclose may be confused about how to provide helpful support and, even though they wish to be supportive, their behaviour may be perceived to be unhelpful (Hays et al. 1994).

The creation and maintenance of a dangerous – or non-dangerous – identity among PHAs and the demographic or individual factors that enable or promote certain kinds of identification, and certain kinds of disclosure patterns, are key areas of inquiry in this volume. The effects of having a dangerous identity on people's navigation of the landscape of social risk and the ways in which it enables or blocks psychological well being also are of great interest to us. We ask what does it mean, socially, to have HIV? We also ask whether PHAs' interpretations of the ramifications of positive serostatus for social support are realistic. These issues are examined in depth after we provide a full description of the settings for the research and the methods for data collection and analysis.

Notes

1 Adam (1998), who has shown how industrialization encouraged a mind-set in which this conceptualization of risk makes sense, also argues that Beck's conceptualization of the 'risk society' is wrong-headed. The notion of risk generally "implies the potential for decisions and calculations" (p. 36), which is not present in relation to environmental hazards. Adam goes so far as to call ours a 'hazard society'. The term 'hazard' implies no sense of choice or calculability: one takes risks, Adam writes, but one does not take hazards – rather, one faces or is threatened by them (pp. 82–83). Despite Adam's insights into the shortcomings of the term 'risk' as Beck uses it, risk rhetoric – and the assumptions regarding calculation and choice that go with it – is dominant today. We therefore satisfy ourselves in using Beck's phrase to describe the current state of affairs in relation to uncertainty and threat.

2 It has been demonstrated that an emphasis on individual culpability diverts attention from the structural causes of ill health (e.g. Balshem 1993; Singer *et al.* 1992; Lupton 1993).

3 In *Choosing Unsafe Sex* (1995b), Sobo demonstrates that women who risk condomless sex gain in status and self-esteem.

Chapter 4

Settings and methods

The research: an overview

The largest data set drawn on in this book was collected between 1991 and 1993 by Green in Scotland and included interviews with PHAs and a seronegative control group. Green's study used a combination of qualitative and quantitative methods, actualized in semi-structured interviews as well as structured questionnaires. Two smaller studies were conducted by Sobo, one in Southern New Mexico in 1993–94 (which used both group and individual interviews) and the other in North-East England in 1996 (which used individual interviews only). A comparison of the methods used and the samples recruited in each site are presented in Tables 4.1 and 4.2 overleaf.

Scotland: the PHA study

The research in Scotland was carried out with PHAs living in the central belt of Scotland, a largely lowland area that includes the country's largest towns and cities (Glasgow and Edinburgh). Three-quarters of the country's five million people live there. The economy, traditionally based on mining, shipbuilding and other heavy industry, is now more dependent on the high technology and service sectors. Unemployment remains relatively high and the social and environmental conditions

Table 4.1 Methods used in each site

	Scotland PHAs	Scotland seronegatives	New Mexico	North-East England
Main approach	Repeated semi-structured qualitative interviews; some quantitative measures	Structured quantitative interviews	Focus group discussion and in-depth semi-structured qualitative interviews	Repeated semi-structured qualitative interviews
Sampling technique	Purposive	Purposive	Purposive	Convenience
Sampling frame	All HIV-positive people living in the central belt of Scotland and accessing services	All people who had tested seronegative living in the central belt of Scotland	All HIV-positive people on the rolls of Las Cruces, New Mexico's 2 HIV/AIDS service centres	All HIV-positive people living in or near Durham County, England, and accessing services
Access	Via gatekeepers at institutions in the area in contact with PHAs	Via gatekeepers at institutions in the area which offered HIV testing	By mail, with a letter documenting the service centres' support of the project	Via the gatekeepers at area HIV/AIDS service centres and via print media (e.g. posters and post cards) displayed in these centres
Number of contacts	1–3 times	Once	1–2 times	3 times
Main topics covered in qualitative interviews (and relevant to this book)	Social support; self-disclosure of serostatus; reactions to disclosure; experience of stigma; reaction to testing positive		Self-disclosure of serostatus; post-test sexual or romantic relationships or experiences	Reaction to testing positive; self-disclosure of serostatus; post-test sexual or romantic relationships or experiences
Quantitative measures collected	Social interaction; social support; demographic and serostatus data	Social interaction; social support; demographic and serostatus data	Demographic and serostatus data only	Demographic and serostatus data only

Table 4.2 The sample(s) in each site[1]

	Scotland PHAs	Scotland seronegatives	New Mexico	North-East England
Total number of respondents	66	67	12	8
Age mean and range	32 (21–49)	30 (18–50)	late 20s to mid-40s[2]	28 (16–33)[3]
Sex:				
Male	54 (81.8%)	56 (82.1%)	7	8
Female	12 (18.2%)	12 (17.9%)	5	
Transmission/Risk group:				
Drug user	28 (42.2%)	26 (38.8%)	Not asked	
Ex drug user	5 (7.6%)	4 (6.0%)		
Gay man	14 (21.2%)	13 (19.4%)		6
Haemophilia	10 (15.2%)	7 (10.4%)		
Other	9 (13.6%)	17 (25.5%)		2
Ethnicity:				
White	66	67	4	8
Black			2	
Hispanic			5	
Asian			1	
Net income (mean) per month[4]	Not asked	Not asked	$563 (£375)	$332 (£498)
HIV-status at first interview:				
AIDS	9 (13.6%)		6	1
HIV+	57 (86.4%)		6	7
Negative	–	67 (100%)		
Educational qualifications			Not asked	Not asked
Yes	32 (48.5%)	39 (58.2%)		
None	34 (51.5%)	28 (41.8%)		
Current residence at first interview:				
Community	48 (72.7%)	49 (73.1%)	12	8
Prison	13 (19.7%)	14 (20.9%)		
Other institution	5 (7.6%)	4 (6%)		
Conjugality:				
Partnered	31 (47%)	33 (49.3%)	6	3
Single	31 (47%)	34 (50.7%)	6	5
Don't know	4 (6%)			

1 We provide no percentages for the New Mexico and North-East England numbers as they are so small; we wish to avoid implying that comparisons can be made, as they cannot.
2 There were so few people with HIV in the area at the time that the data were collected that to be any more specific than this might violate our promise of anonymity.
3 Generally, nobody under the age of 18 would have been included in the research. However, the 16-year-old was sent by a social worker and his age was only found to be 16 after he already was involved in the study. As his participation was voluntary, as his social worker supported it, and as his participation did not conflict with departmental research ethics rulings on the work, he was not eliminated. The median age was 28, as was the mean when the youth's age was removed from the equation.
4 Our conversion rate is 1.5 dollars to the pound, which was typical in the early 1990s.

in the least-favoured areas account for the fact that Scottish children face one of the highest risks of growing up in poverty in the European Union (Scottish Council Foundation 1998). The peripheral housing schemes surrounding the cities became known in the 1980s as centres of British drug culture. The central belt as a whole, however, is famous for its natural beauty and also includes affluent suburban and rural areas.

At the time of the research, about 2000 people in Scotland had been diagnosed as seropositive. Current figures show that of the 2733 HIV-positive people living in Scotland 42 per cent were infected through IDU practices (compared to only 8 per cent of cases reported elsewhere in the UK). Other infection groups are men who had sex with men (32%), those infected heterosexually (18%), those infected by blood or tissue transfer (4%), and those with other or undetermined modes of infection (4%) (PHLS AIDS Centre 1998). Ninety per cent of Scotland's HIV-infected residents live in the central belt, mostly in the cities Glasgow and Edinburgh.

The study sample was theoretical, or 'purposive': while sample members were not selected at random, considerable care was taken to include members of all transmission groups and to recruit from a variety of settings, thus maximizing the representativeness of the group. This approach was necessitated by the difficulty we would have had in recruiting participants in a truly random fashion. The numbers of PHAs were too low for successful random sampling.

Further, while fear of participating in an 'AIDS study' may not be seen in larger, more cosmopolitan areas, the populations of both Glasgow and Edinburgh are each less than one million; each has fairly small and concentrated gay and drug using communities. Even in 1991–93, the stigma attached to AIDS made recruitment extremely difficult, despite the good connections that Green had established through the Medical Research Council (MRC) and various AIDS service groups and providers.

Recruitment was carried out in diverse settings including outpatient clinics, prisons, drug rehabilitation units, general practices, and through self-help and voluntary support organizations. The recruitment procedure varied in each setting according to the advice and requirements of the 'gatekeepers' in each organization that allowed us access. In some settings we were able to recruit directly. More often, however, the gatekeeper arranged a meeting after having obtained consent from a potential participant. All participants gave written consent to participate in the study before being interviewed. Characteristics of the sample are shown in Table 4.2.

The PHAs were interviewed at home, in the researchers' offices, or in the recruitment centre, as each preferred. Interviews took between one and three hours. Both quantitative and qualitative data were collected. Numerical data were collected systematically to provide measures of social network and social support. In addition details of social relationships, disclosure of HIV status and experiences of stigma were discussed at length. Most of the in-depth interviews were audio-taped although not all participants wished to be recorded and taping was not permitted in the interviews conducted in prisons. In these interviews, more extensive notes than usual were taken.

All the PHAs were interviewed by Green or her male colleague Stephen Platt. Participants were allowed to choose the gender of the interviewer, although in practice only one woman expressed a preference.[1] Green and Platt met frequently to check consistency and reliability, and exchanged interview schedules, transcripts and notes.

Members of the sample were visited annually three times over a three-year period. Of the 66 people initially interviewed 46 were interviewed at least once more and 28 were interviewed three times. The main cause of loss to follow-up was death; almost one-third of the sample died during the course of the study. Also, a high proportion of the prisoners were lost to follow-up on their release from prison, and some of the drug users were lost due to their high mobility.[2]

The aim of the repeat contacts was two-fold: first, to monitor possible changes, and second, to develop more robust relationships with participants to obtain data of greater depth. At each contact, the same quantitative measures were collected and subjects were asked in depth about the same aspects of their social relationships and disclosure.

As Table 4.2 indicates, the majority of the participants were male, reflecting national AIDS statistics, and all were white, reflecting the sparseness of the non-white population of the area. Participants were mostly in their late 20s and early 30s (mean age 32). Representatives of all the main transmission groups were included. Initially, almost one-half of the sample were current or ex-IDUs, but due to a higher rate of attrition among IDUs, the proportion fell to less than one-third in the second interview.

Less than half the participants had any educational qualifications,[3] and the majority had last been employed in manual work in factories, building sites or in the service sector. Many had worked in the informal sector, for example, as labourers, bar workers, prostitutes, 'fences' (people who deal in stolen goods) or drug dealers. The majority were in receipt of welfare benefits and not employed at the time of the interviews. Whilst this was sometimes due to ill health, many were unemployed prior to being diagnosed, usually on account of either drug use or haemophilia. About one-half had a sexual partner; and one-half were single at the time of the first interview. These proportions stayed approximately the same over the course of the study.

At first contact, the majority were asymptomatic, but 17 (26%) had experienced quite definite symptoms of HIV disease and 9 (14%) had AIDS. The mean year of diagnosis of seropositivity (collected at first contact in 1991) was 1987 (range 1983–91), and most participants had been living with HIV for several years.

Quantitative measures and analysis: PHAs and seronegatives compared

In order to provide data with which to compare the social relationships of the PHAs, we recruited a sample of people who had tested seronegative. The seronegative participants were broadly matched with the PHA sample for age, gender, education status and risk group membership. They were recruited from the same hospital clinics and prisons as the HIV-positive sample and were all living in the central belt of Scotland, the great majority in Glasgow or Edinburgh.[4]

The following measures were collected from both sets of participants to enable comparison of the social networks and social support of both groups (discussed in Chapter 11). All were constructed specifically for this study as other measures designed for use with PHAs and available at that time (e.g. Namir *et al.* 1989a, 1989b; Zich and Temoshok 1987; Martin and Dean 1988) would not have been sufficiently specific to the needs of participants in our sample. Few of our participants, for example, were regularly asked to dinner parties or had a need for someone to water their houseplants when they were out of town (two questions asked to measure social support among gay men in the USA).

Our first measure, derived from a social contact list, was designed to provide a relatively objective indication of social contact. Participants were asked to list all the people with whom they had frequent contact in the last month or who were important or particularly close to them. Then, they were asked to say how often they had contact with each person on the list. From this, a measure of *sociability* was derived: the higher the score, the greater the frequency of contact with people in their social network. From the social contact list we were also able to examine and compare the composition of the social network; that is, we were able to define proportions of *kin, friends* and *professional contacts*. Contacts who had been lost in the previous year or with whom the participant had had less-than-frequent contact were also listed to provide a measure of *lost contact*.

Social support was measured in a number of ways to ensure each aspect and domain of such support that we considered important in light of the literature was covered. We asked questions covering three domains of support (social interaction, material and emotional support). Each question was delivered in three parts to find out whether this support had actually been received in the last three months; if not, whether it was perceived as available; and whether the participant was satisfied with this level of support. From the answers, we calculated measures of *actual* and *perceived social interaction, material support*, and *emotional support* and *satisfaction* levels, as well as a *total social support score*.

Another measure was an assessment of the existence of, and support from, confidants, as this source of support is said to be particularly important for people with chronic illness (Wortman 1984). Participants were asked to assess on a Likert-type scale six dimensions of confidant support that they had access to (do you have people who: understand you well; you can tell your worries to; share their problems with you; you feel relaxed with; are available when you need them; comfort you). A cumulative *confidant scale* was constructed from these responses, a higher score indicating greater support.

The final measure of support was constructed from participants' assessment, on another Likert-type scale, of six dimensions of stress resulting from contact with people providing social support (are there people who: ask for more than they offer in return; you argue with; make you feel bad; are difficult to talk to about HIV/AIDS; you worry about; make unreasonable demands). A cumulative *social stress scale* was constructed from these responses, a higher score indicating greater social stress.

Other variables that are used in the analysis include: *age; gender; sexual orientation* (whether the participant self-reported as gay or heterosexual); *drug use* (whether or not the participant had injected drugs or been using methadone in the last six months); *haemophilia; prisoner status* (yes or no).

Data were analyzed using the Statistical Package for Social Sciences (SPSS for Windows Version 6.1, 1995). T-tests were used to compare the scores of seropositives and seronegatives on the social network and social support measures. T-tests and analysis of variance were used to compare scores of men and women, and different groups of PHAs.

Las Cruces, New Mexico study of PHAs

Las Cruces is a small, economically poor, relatively conservative one-mall desert town in Southern New Mexico. Southern New Mexico is a rural region with low population density. While New Mexico had reported a total of 861 AIDS cases by the end of 1993, only 81 of those came from Southern counties. Only 32 came from the Las Cruces region (*New Mexico HIV Disease Update* 1994: 10).

Even now, very little research has been carried out with rural US PHAs, whose needs may differ greatly from those of the cosmopolitan populations more commonly investigated, such as in New York, Miami, San Francisco, and London. The research conducted in Las Cruces in 1994 aimed, ultimately, to help fill this gap; its immediate aim was to generate a set of guidelines for successful self-disclosure strategies that local AIDS counsellors could share with clients.

The study was based at two Las Cruces agencies offering services to PHAs. Although a purposive sampling strategy was followed, because of small numbers the sample assembled was, essentially, a convenience sample. Recruitment was carried out by mail. Each of the two agencies' 68 local area clients was sent a small packet containing a letter explaining the plan – and the need – for the study, contact information, and a brief demographic survey.[5]

The response rate was 37 per cent (n = 25). This is favourable when compared with general response rates of between 20 and 25 per cent for the regional agency's survey mailings (T. Call, personal communication, 1993). Of the 25 individuals in total who responded, just under half (n = 12) were able to participate. Often, non-participation was explained as due to failing health; the idiom of health may be useful for persons not wishing to talk about their condition for other reasons.

The study originally called for focus groups only. Three men and five women participated in focus groups, two of which were held. Four individuals could or would not attend the focus groups but wanted to help with the research. To allow them a chance to participate, and to collect further information from three focus-group participants who also expressed interest in being interviewed individually, seven private interviews were arranged. They were carried out by Sobo and graduate [UK: post-graduate] student Jude Drapeau (both white women). The concerns of the four interview-only participants were found similar to those of both the five focus-group-only and the three focus-group-and-interview participants.

The sample is described in Table 4.2 on p. 47. It consisted of five women and seven men. Ages ranged from late 20s to mid-40s. The average monthly income (after taxes) was $562.75 (about £375). Half of the participants had AIDS.

Every effort was made to ensure from the outset that all risk groups were represented but, on the advice of service workers involved in recruitment efforts, in order to avoid offending participants, mode of transmission was not formally ascertained. Notwithstanding, during the course of the research, it became clear that the majority of the seven men believed they were infected through sex with other men. Drug use also may have been a vector: two of the seven men and three of the five women volunteered that they were ex-IDUs. And at least two of the five women were infected during heterosexual intercourse, one by her estranged, bisexual husband.

The focus groups met at agency offices in the early evenings, after hours. Copies of the mailed information letter and demographic survey were provided. Informed consent was verbally given. Discussions were audio-taped, with permission, and participants were paid $20 (about £13) for their time. The same procedures were followed with interviewees, who were interviewed at their convenience, in locations of their own choosing (generally, their homes).

One of the reasons for holding focus groups when in-depth ethnographic research is impossible is to allow the ethnographer access to detailed narrative data concerning intersubjectively held understandings regarding a given topic (see Schwartz 1978). Such data bespeak key dimensions of the intracultural debate surrounding the topic under question and provide information as to the dialogical contexts in which specific kinds of responses will be provoked. These dimensions, which Sobo has called "nodes of contention" (Sobo 1995a), may be particularly apparent when heterogeneous groups are assembled.

Indeed, in this case the mix of participants was beneficial: difference moved people to ask questions of others and make distinctions and clarifications in the focus groups that they might otherwise not have seen the need for (see Bender and Ewbank 1994; *cf.* VanLandingham *et al.* 1994). Focus groups have been shown to have "great potential" for AIDS research, in part because they can be "uniquely effective in obtaining information from hard-to-reach populations" (Shedlin and Schreiber 1994: 17) such as the ones this research concerns. Moreover, they only call for a small sample, such as this research used.

Audio-tapes were transcribed, and Sobo performed an iterative content analysis to identify salient themes and narrative patterns. Particular attention was paid to situational contexts that block or enable self-disclosure, successful and unsuccessful self-disclosure strategies, and moralizing rhetoric.

North-East England study of PHAs

The research in England's North-East was initiated in response to discussions undertaken in 1995 with members of Cleveland County's Social Services and Research and Intelligence units.[6] The project was based in County Durham, but participants also came from the counties of Tyne and Wear, to the north, and Cleveland, to the south. These counties, north of Yorkshire and south of Northumberland and the Scottish border, are among the most impoverished in England, their once strong heavy industries of shipbuilding, mining, and steel production having crumbled in the face of Thatcherite policies and foreign competition in the early 1980s.

Initially, participant recruitment was facilitated by three individuals affiliated with local hospital outpatient clinics and social service organizations. Starting in February, 1996, gatekeepers at these sites forwarded project information packets to clients and associates.

While local interest in and support for the research from AIDS activists and service professionals was very high, recruitment was problematic. This was partly due to the small number of HIV-positive people in the area. By March 31 1994, only 405 people in the North had tested positive for HIV.[7] Only 141 people had been diagnosed with AIDS; 99 of whom had already died. The Local [Health] Authorities expected that actual figures were between 12–31 per cent higher than reported figures (McManus 1994).

When several months passed with only four volunteers coming forward, recruitment efforts were expanded by distributing brightly coloured posters, flyers, and postcards describing the project to AIDS activists and self-help and voluntary support organizations. After this recruitment strategy had been in place for three months, four more volunteers had come forth. Recruitment efforts ceased at this point. The resultant sample of eight men is described in Table 4.2 (on p. 47).

Participants were provided with an information sheet that began with a brief informed consent statement. The statement explained the interview process and, in common with the other studies described above, emphasized participants' right to withdraw from the study at any time, and promised confidentiality and anonymity. Consent was verbal.

The questionnaire topics were adapted from the New Mexico study. Data gathered from social and health service gatekeepers in the initial project planning stage were used to make culturally-sensitive local adjustments. More importantly, stereotypes related to AIDS were included as a topic, reflecting Sobo's growing interest in identity in relation to positive HIV test results.

Sobo and Paula Black, an advanced (ABD) sociology graduate [UK: post-graduate] student, carried out the interviews. Both are white, as were all the interviewees, but while Sobo is from the USA, Black is from the UK. Interview meetings were arranged at the convenience of the participants and took place in locations of their choosing. Transportation costs were reimbursed, and participants were paid £15 (about $23) for each interview.

Sessions were audio-taped with permission; interviewers also took notes related to what was said and the interview environment. Each participant undertook three interviews with the same interviewer, except two, who were unable to schedule a final appointment within the time-frame available to the interviewers.

Interviews were transcribed, and Sobo performed an iterative content analysis to identify salient themes and narrative patterns. Particular attention was paid to situational contexts that block or enable self-disclosure, successful and unsuccessful self-disclosure strategies, and stereotypes and their ramifications for living with HIV.

Limitations and linkages

Each of the studies described above has certain limitations. Most importantly, none boasts a truly random or representative sample. Whilst attempts were made to maximize the groups represented in each sample, each study sample was essentially self-selected, limiting the generalizability of our findings: the participants may differ systematically from PHAs who did not volunteer to participate. This may have introduced certain biases into the data. Persons responding to the call to participate acknowledge their seropositivity and feel willing to discuss their private concerns with, or in front of, a stranger.

Confidentiality was a concern of many subjects in all three studies and deterred a number of those approached from participating. It was a central concern in Las Cruces and the North-East of England. HIV-positive citizens in non-urban areas may understandably fear having relatives, neighbours, or co-workers see them enter offices associated in the public's mind with AIDS or, for that matter, university-linked endeavours. In Glasgow, being seen with Green was a possible source of similar anxiety, as Green had become known to a section of the drug-using population as 'the woman who wants to talk to people with HIV'. The perceived threats of participating in an AIDS-related project in such social circumstances, despite the promise of confidentiality and anonymity, must be intense (see also Laryea and Gien 1993).

Some of the limitations related to sample size and shape were site specific. By the end of year three, the number of participants in the Scottish study was down to 28, which limited the scope of longitudinal quantitative analysis. The Southern New Mexico and North-East England samples were very small from the outset – although the populations they were drawn from were very small too. While small samples may not hinder qualitative analysis so long as sufficient data redundancy occurs prior to ending recruitment – and we feel it did – quantitative analysis with small samples is problematic. Because of this, in both the latter cases, no statistical or quantitative analyses based on sample size have been undertaken. To do so would be to misrepresent the findings and to distort their significance.

Recruitment efforts were confined to adults over the age of 18.[8] We therefore do not address issues specific to youths with HIV, and the findings we present from our samples may not be pertinent to this younger age group.

To generalize from the qualitative findings also would be perilous. The narratives provide rich, evocative descriptions of what the experience of being HIV positive in certain circumstances can be like for certain individuals. The familiarity of each individual's stories when compared with the stories told by the rest, both within and across sample groups, suggests that similar experiences may be commonplace for many. Many of the factors that shape PHAs' experiences may be artifacts of a shared culture – a global Western culture – rather than unique to each site. But because our samples were small and non-random, we have no scientific justification for such a claim.

Another sample-related limitation is specific to the focus group method. Focus groups cannot be used to measure real-life levels of cultural consensus. Rather, they are designed to identify and explore some of the culturally charged issues around which agreement or disagreement can turn.

A second limitation of the focus groups convened in New Mexico was linked to the limited number of HIV-positive people in Las Cruces: some of the focus group participants knew each other already. This may have promoted self-protective secrecy; it also may have kept the involved participants from spinning tales and may have led them to introduce certain topics for discussion that otherwise might have been neglected (at times, for example, one person would correct the other or ask a specific question of her or him).

Because social context has a strong influence on the ways in which people present themselves to others and to themselves, the identities projected in any of our focus group discussions or individual interviews were necessarily partial. In individual interviews, subjects may tell the interviewer what they think s/he wants to hear. In a focus group the contrived and public nature of the undertaking may intensify the effects of particular social and cultural constraints, including ideas about what constitutes acceptable group behaviour. An ethnographic grasp of the cultural context is therefore essential for the productive use of both focus group and individual interview data.

Moreover, the stories we were told are individual recreations of reality, which may have little or no correspondence to actual behaviours or events. Therefore, we can report from focus group and interview data only on the subjective construction of social reality. And because the construction is, in many cases, retrospective, reliability in the best of circumstances is only as good as participants' memories. People are likely to retain selectively the most extreme experiences; further, felt stigma will bias accounts. Negative incidents may well be wrongly attributed by participants to their HIV status. From qualitative interview and focus group data, we can therefore only report on what people *say* they do or feel or have experienced, not what they actually do feel or have gone through.

In addition to sample-related shortcomings, and the particular shortcomings of the interview and focus group techniques, the research also is limited by the fact that the three studies reported here were not conceived as one at origin. There are marked differences between them. The in-depth qualitative methods used differed in each regional setting, as did the locations used for data collection. Moreover, the quantitative data collected, demographics included, differed at each site.

The original aims of the three studies were distinct as were the local needs they contrived to meet, and the content of the interviews therefore varied. While the central focus at all sites involved social relationships, interviews at each site approached these from a different angle. Discussion in Scotland was all-encompassing whereas self-disclosure to sexual partners in New Mexico and identity in North-East England took the main stage. Moreover, the Scottish study included quantitative data to compare PHAs to a matched seronegative group. No such data were collected in New Mexico or North-East England.

Methodological differences notwithstanding, a grounded theory approach guided data collection and analysis at each site. Models were developed in intimate relationship with the data as it was collected (see Glaser and Strauss 1968b).

Strength in numbers?

Despite the potential confusion that might arise in our attempt at discussing results from three studies in one book, there are important advantages to our undertaking. The range of methods and samples serves to maximize the validity of our findings, as a type of methodological triangulation. HIV is, worldwide, a life-threatening virus for which there is no known cure. It seems likely that a type of experience or under-standing reported by a drug user interviewed in Scotland that is reiterated by a gay black man in a focus group in New Mexico and a straight white man in England may be generalizable to other PHAs in the USA and the UK.

Further, while many studies of PHAs tend to focus on one risk group, mostly gay men, the studies reported here include mixed samples in terms of transmission mode, sexuality, and gender (Scotland); ethnicity, gender, and sexuality (New Mexico); and sexuality (England). This enables us to draw the experiences of a range of people from diverse backgrounds into our analysis. It allows us to identify some of the similarities and differences that being a PHA in the Western world entails.

Despite interesting regional variations and local quirks, the people of all three locations participate, albeit to varying degrees, in a global Western culture that villifies HIV and constructs HIV-positive people as criminal, immoral, or at least dangerous beings. It is against this background that careful generalizations can be made. One of the factors that will affect the generalizability of findings is the cosmopolitan nature of the site to which one wishes to extend them; all of our sites were limited in this respect. Further, as will be discussed in later chapters, certain demographic factors, such as whether a person is gay and whether s/he belongs to a strong community of similar individuals, may be crucial in fostering the inter-nalization of a negative – or a positive – HIV identity or identity dimension. These factors also affect one's experience of and attitude toward HIV infection and AIDS-related disease as well as AIDS-related risk-taking (e.g. Quimby 1992; Sobo 1995b, 1997; Ward 1993a). But, local differences notwithstanding, the concerns related to social relationships, social risk, and stigma that were expressed in all three sites were often extremely similar, and we believe that we have as much to learn from this fact as we do from the differences that have been recorded.

The experiences of the participants at the three sites overlapped so much that, were it not for our use of standard record-keeping procedures from the start of this joint project (precisely labeling data sources, etc.), we might easily have mistaken findings from one site for findings generated at another. Examples in the chapters to follow amply demonstrate this fact. To assist the reader (and ourselves) we present findings from each site separately, and when that is not desirable we identify the geographic location of each respondent quoted. We quote from representative testimony recorded at one site in the midst of presenting findings from another only where doing so adds to the picture we strive to present and augments the model we attempt to put forward. Our practice of identifying sources allows the reader to draw his or her own conclusions about the extent to which our findings are replicated at each site.

We illustrate many of the key concepts through the use of quotations from participants, because our empirical focus is the perceptions of people with HIV. As others have done before (e.g. Robinson 1990; Williams 1984), we use narratives to promote an understanding of the experience of chronic illness. Participants' own first-hand reports contain a depth of feeling and knowledge that our authorial voice can only partially and distortedly convey. In the end, it is by disseminating PHAs' stories in their own words that we will attain the main goal of our studies. To this end we present to the reader a vivid account of the ways that PHAs report coping with the stigma associated with AIDS and the manner in which the disease is perceived as vastly altering their everyday social interactions.

Notes

1   This enabled Green and Platt to reflect upon the possible impact of same- and other-gender interviewing, and may have added to the breadth of the data collected: many participants seemed to feel comfortable talking about different aspects of their lives according to whether they were being interviewed by a same- or other-gender interviewer.

2   People living at participant-provided contact addresses often claimed not to know the whereabouts of the participant, and due to the confidential nature of the study we were unwilling to probe further.

3   That is, they left school at the age of 16 without passing any of the national examinations leading to recognized qualifications.

4   We had no access to medical records of any kind to check the seronegativity of respondents but relied on the assessment of gatekeepers at the various recruitment sites. This was then checked further with participants during the interview who were asked during the course of the interview about their experience of testing negative.

5   Sobo prepared the mailings but did not mail them; that task was left to an agency staff member who had access to the roster and so could make mailing labels without compromising the anonymity and confidentiality concerns of the clients. Sobo explained this process to clients in the letter so that they would know that she did not have access to their contact information.

6   Sobo was put in contact with HIV Coordinator Jim McManus after this event, and his support was invaluable. Cleveland County has since been disbanded.

7   This figure represents cases reported in the former Northern Regional Health Authority area, and not just in the North-East. In the mid-90s, the Health Authorities and certain counties in England were reorganized. Therefore, figures for the specific area of interest are not always grouped as we would have them.

8   Only adults were recruited by the researchers. However, one participant's age was found to be 16 after he already was involved in the study. As his participation was voluntary, as his social worker sent him to us, and as his participation did not conflict with departmental research ethics rulings, he was not eliminated.

Chapter 5

Living with HIV: coping with a new status

The HIV test

The necessity of 'the test'

Receiving a positive HIV antibody test result generally is a prerequisite for adopting an identity that entails HIV. But a positive test is not sufficient cause to do so and it also is not always necessary. Some people may know they are HIV positive because of their symptoms and sometimes these, or having had a lover (or injecting partner) who also was seropositive, provide proof enough. Medical confirmation of what they know to be true is not seen as necessary[1] (*cf.* Huby 1999; Lindenbaum and Lock 1993). And then there are others who consciously make fake claims to AIDS.

Both authors have heard rumours about HIV-negative people who adopt (or seek to adopt) AIDS identities in order to gain health and welfare benefits, or pity, or entry into a study for which they will be paid incentive fees (*cf.* Strauss *et al.* 1992). Some are said to fake seropositivity in order to terrify those who might otherwise exert power over them, such as police officers or sexual partners; others are said to do it to shame passers-by or even close relations into providing handouts.

While we did not specifically ask about fake PHAs, two of the eight participants in the North-East England sample spontaneously mentioned people close to them who had made false claims to having been 'diagnosed'. For example, Bob, a heterosexual ex-warehouseman said that his gay cousin falsely told his family that he 'was HIV'.

> and everyone hit the roof. ..."Do you know he is dying, do you know he has got six months left?" I went "Now hold on a minute. I know he is gay but how long ago did he say to you that he has only got six months?" "Oh a few months back." I went "Oh, right." So I went up to see him. ...I said "I thought you were dying." ...He said "Well I am going." ... He was going on because he was gay, he wanted sympathy ... he thought that everyone was going to feel sorry for him but he had a shock when I came up and dragged him out of [a disco], stuck him in the car and drove him all the way down to [town] for him to apologize to the family.

Another participant, Jamie, who is gay, described what happened with a not-too-close friend of his:

> [Gary] informed me that he was HIV positive himself but something at the back of my mind didn't gel and he had a very, very, very, very close female friend and we both talked and we both said the same thing that we thought that – we didn't want to turn round and call [Gary] a liar but something wasn't right. He had no contact with Dr. Snow, with Ward 25 [to whom, and where, PHAs in the area would go, and] there was just something wrong somewhere and it was to do with [Gary's] alcoholism really it was part of his cry for attention and for help and for people to pity him, it was something to make him important in other people's eyes.

In both cases, we cannot know whether the accusations of falsity are true in any objective sense. Jamie did say of his friend that "when he was drunk he once told me that he wasn't HIV. ...He said that they had confused his name with someone else who lived in the same block of flats but at a different number, which is a very lame sort of excuse to try and pull." This did not suggest to Jamie, but did suggest to us, the possibility that Gary's confession may itself have been a form of denial on the part of a man who actually was HIV positive; that is, it may have been an effort at normalization – a strategy that we explore later. Jamie's desire to dismiss his friend's claim to be seropositive, and Bob's dismissal of his cousin's story, may have had as much to do with the stress of keeping their own seropositivity under wraps, or possibly even a complex feeling of being upstaged, as it had with the actuality of the other men's seronegative status. Whatever the objective reality in these stories, both illustrate the intense impact of claiming an HIV identity.

Getting tested

While a study of the veracity of these types of narratives and of the social, cultural and psychological processes underlying the generation and spread of what we'll call 'AIDS Imposter Tales' would make for fascinating reading, here we have only sufficient space (and data) to discuss the adoption of AIDS identities by truly seropositive people.[2] And seropositivity means testing positive for antibodies to HIV, the virus associated with AIDS.

According to CDC estimates, about half of all US PHAs do not know they have been infected (Levi 1996). The US National AIDS Behavioral Survey found that more than 60 per cent of those at the highest risk for infection had not been tested for HIV antibodies (Berrios *et al.* 1993: 1579). Many people at risk do not perceive themselves as such and so do not get tested; in one US study, serotesting only those inner-city women who perceived themselves as being at risk would have left un-detected as much as 70 per cent of all seropositivity in the sample (Lindsay *et al.* 1989).

Barriers to HIV test uptake notwithstanding, results take anything from 24 hours to two weeks to be returned. The period between having one's blood drawn and finding out if one is or is not HIV positive can be trying (regarding the initial decision to get tested and the pros and cons of testing itself, see Bor *et al.* 1991; Coates *et al.* 1988; Meadows *et al.* 1990; Sobo 1994). Many test-takers do not return to the test site to find out their results; at CDC-funded sites, only 60 per cent of those tested come back (Levi 1996).

Those who do return often find the vocabulary that clinicians use to talk about the test confusing, which can lead to misinterpretations of results. For instance, a Scottish participant with haemophilia was told his result was "positive" and he at first interpreted this as meaning 'good' and that he was free from infection. Further, as Kurth and Hutchinson (1989) point out, people who think that they have 'passed' the HIV test sometimes equate their perceived negativity with immunity, and this can lead to an attitude of complacency or even to an increase in risk behaviour (*cf.* Kinsey 1994).[3]

Testing Positive: Stages of Adjustment

If test results are positive, the person must adjust to his or her new status as a PHA.[4] Participants often spoke as if infection with HIV is a state of being: 'He's not HIV', 'I'm HIV', 'When you're HIV'. HIV becomes as much an identifier as religion

('She's Jewish'), nationality ('He's American'), and other identity components. In contrast, people 'have AIDS' – they do not become it.

Most research on adjustment to positive test results concerns homo- or bisexual men who belong to relatively organized urban gay communities. Working with mostly homosexual men, McCain and Gramling (1992) identified three separate phases of seropositivity or AIDS coping. These processual phases were (a) Living with Dying (b) Fighting the Sickness, and (c) Getting Worn Out. 'Living with Dying' begins with a positive diagnosis and the initial desire to deny it and the death that, sooner or later, it brings. The desire to deny is not limited to non-heterosexual men: for example, denial as well as related pathological behaviours, such as increased drug use, are especially likely among substance-using women (Kurth and Hutchinson 1989). Denial is also more common among Black HIV-positive gay men (Leserman *et al.* 1992). For some people, denial persists even as symptoms of AIDS develop (Earl *et al.* 1991–92).

Intuitively, denial seems a counter-productive response. It is true that it may be correlated with higher levels of sexual risk taking (e.g. Joseph *et al.* 1989). But, as Joseph *et al.* point out, "There is a growing appreciation for the role of denial or illusion in the maintenance of psychological functioning" (p. 211); denial can contribute to "a robust sense of psychological well being" (p. 211). Those who engage in the strategy of denial may have lower emotional stress levels than those who do not deny the correctness of their diagnoses.

Beyond the urge to deny – an urge that may be dodged or succumbed to – 'Living with Dying' also entails "anger, depression, suicidal ideation, and fear of rejection by others" (McCain and Gramling 1992: 276). Sleep and communication disorders, increased anxiety, and hypochondria also have been observed. Women who test positive may feel overcome by guilt about their possible roles as transmitters of HIV to their children.[5] They are also probably as likely as closeted or self-loathing homosexual men to "experience feelings of overwhelming shame" (Kurth and Hutchinson 1989: 262) as a result of their seropositivity. It may be taken to signal their participation in socially unacceptable practices (e.g. illicit drug use, multiple casual sexual relations, a relationship with a man who is unfaithful). Whether female or male, PHAs who feel stigmatized may also feel unable to inform members of their social networks of their condition. This can lead to "increased isolation during a time of great need" (p. 262).

Moving from the anger and fear of the first phase of coping into the next, 'Fighting the Sickness', involves making the decision to, as McCain and Gramling say, "get on with one's life" (1992: 278). Social network membership shifts as rejecting individuals drop out, as those deemed somehow threatening (e.g. as hateful, accusing, or merely unsupportive) are avoided, and as more HIV-positive individuals are incorporated.[6]

Such incorporation, of course, depends on the density of PHAs in the area, and the extent to which one identifies with them. While urban gay men may have no problem skewing membership in their networks toward PHAs, people in rural areas may not know other PHAs with whom they might socialize. And a homophobic heterosexual may not wish to associate with other PHAs if most are gay. But people 'Fighting the Sickness' focus not just on locating and cultivating friendships with supportive people. They also have concrete physical goals such as getting enough rest and eating well.

While 'Fighting the Sickness' often involves purposeful health-seeking behaviour, financial and other needs may thwart this, as might gender expectations. For example, poorer seropositive women who would like to nurture themselves often cannot because of material and social obstacles such as money shortages, familial responsibilities, and the classism, sexism, and racism built into the health care delivery system (Hutchinson 1993; Ward 1993a). Further, impoverished people and those not deemed 'at risk' often are not diagnosed until AIDS has overtaken them (Kurth and Hutchinson 1989). It is quite possible that members of these groups move through the 'Fighting the Sickness' phase much faster than McCain and Gramling's mostly gay male sample did before proceeding into the final stage, in which death is no longer fought.

While McCain and Gramling identified stages of coping, much of the literature on 'living with HIV' identifies 'themes' instead. Barroso (1997), for example, identifies five dimensions of coping for a sample of 14 men and 6 women with AIDS: normalizing, focusing on living, taking care of oneself, being in relation to others, and triumphing. These dimensions represent "not a linear process but an overlapping whole" (p. 63).

Coping strategies help people to cope with specific challenges. Siegel and Krauss (1991) identify three major adaptive challenges faced by their sample of 55 seropositive gay men. These include dealing with the possibility of a curtailed life span, dealing with reactions to a stigmatizing illness, and developing strategies for maintaining physical and emotional health. Notwithstanding, they note that these challenges "are likely to change or to assume different priorities as [people] encounter the more or less manageable manifestations of HIV disease" (p. 26).

So, PHA's engagement level with each of Siegel and Krauss's challenges will ebb and flow, just as Barroso's coping strategies overlap. In other words, while it is helpful to conceptualize adjustment to seropositivity as a series of stages, progression is not always linear and a palate of coping mechanisms may be selected from as challenges surface and recede. It is therefore more helpful to think of adjustment to

HIV as a process, rather than as a series of static states being entered into after passing digital thresholds of some kind. Further, it may be that while crisis-type thresholds exist that amplify certain aspects of HIV's impact, after they pass people can return to a steady state rather than always having to progress to a different stage of adjustment.

Psychological adjustment[7]

Is there a verdict?

For most PHAs, diagnosis is associated with a dramatic curtailment of life expectancy and on-going physical deterioration. This itself can entail a great psychological burden. So can other features of the disease, such as its stigma, its implications for identity, uncertainty about the onset and nature of symptoms, uncertainty about the way one will respond to treatment (as well as when or if to begin it).

All told, it is not surprising that many assume that an HIV-positive diagnosis has a detrimental impact upon psychological health. But published research in this area has not presented consistent results. This is at least partly due to the use of a variety of incompatible, unstandardized measures and a tendency for samples to be small and comprised of one 'risk group' (see Green et al. 1996; Dew et al. 1997). Furthermore, literature in this area is, at present, almost exclusively based on research that was conducted prior to the widespread use of combination therapies, which have extended the life expectancy of some PHAs and may have affected the psychosocial impact of diagnosis.

In the main, published research tends to support the hypothesis that seropositive people have poorer psychological health than seronegatives (e.g. Catalan et al. 1992a, 1992b; Perkins et al. 1993) and an increased suicide risk (e.g. Cote et al. 1992; Marzuk et al. 1988) – at least at times of crisis. It is unclear, however, whether those PHAs who have poor mental health do so as a result of their diagnosis or because they tend to come from groups that may have poor psychological health to begin with (Platt 1992; Marzuk and Perry 1993; Kelly et al. 1998). And, at least for some members of the white US middle class, positive test results may be interpreted as a blessing, either literally, in a religious sense, or because they have led to a feeling of purpose, or life understanding, that was previously lacking (Stanley 1999; cf. Gatter 1995). Stanley suggests that those who view their seropositive status in this way may be more likely to engage in physically and psychosocially health-promoting behaviour.

Even those studies that report an association between seropositivity and higher psychological distress have found that most seropositive people are free of psychological disorders (Brown and Rundell 1993; Catalan *et al.* 1992a, 1992b; Fell *et al.* 1993; Perry and Fishman 1993). Although psychological disturbance may occur at transitional points in the disease, such as during HIV testing, it does not seem to persist (Perry *et al.* 1990a).

It has been argued that psychological morbidity of PHAs increases with number of physical symptoms and stage of disease, at least among haemophiliacs (Catalan *et al.* 1992a) and gay men (Catalan 1992b; Hays *et al.* 1992; Fell *et al.* 1993; Kessler *et al.* 1988; Ostrow *et al.* 1989). Nonetheless, Rabkin *et al.* (1991, 1997) failed to find an association between disease progression and psychosocial status of seropositive people, and in a study of suicide in long-term AIDS survivors (Rabkin *et al.* 1993) found a high level of positive psychological health independent of HIV illness stage.

Overall, the literature suggests that there are few psychological differences between seropositive and seronegative people and that most people with HIV cope adequately with their illness for much of the time. There may, however, be short periods of psychological disturbance following key crises in the illness such as diagnosis, first offer of treatment, or hospitalization related to HIV (Fell *et al.* 1993). The shock and identity turmoil resulting from a diagnosis, as described in earlier chapters, has been widely reported and in most regions of the USA and the UK a range of counselling services have been set up to provide support (although access can still be an issue). The process of coming to terms with an HIV diagnosis and each new stage in its progression involves a wide range of adjustments and changes (Miller 1987), as does self-reinvention.

Findings from Scotland

Some of the data from Scotland helps to clarify several aspects of the links between psychosocial health and HIV serostatus.[8] The links may have changed somewhat, for some people, in response to the recently extended life expectancy of US and UK PHAs. The research, like the vast bulk of the literature, is based on assumptions of limited life expectancy. Nevertheless, the following résumé of psychosocial adjustment findings from the Scottish study have implications for theories of stigma management and identity construction and maintenance, and the processes entailed for such are not affected by medical breakthroughs. Further, breakthroughs have in some ways made the findings even more compelling as, even prior to the break-throughs and without the hope these may have engendered,[9] psychological well being among Scottish PHAs was, in general, just as good as that of the seronegative controls.

Whilst a few seropositive participants claimed to be "depressed the majority of the time," most said that, although they had experienced periods of psychological disturbance since their diagnosis, they in general felt no more or less disturbed than before diagnosis. Neither were they significantly more anxious nor more depressed nor did they have lower self-esteem than the matched sample of seronegatives, as measured by self-report.

That HIV did not cause the majority of seropositive participants in Scotland to be psychologically disturbed most of the time appeared to be related to the strategies adopted to cope with the illness. The long-term nature of HIV disease and the relative healthiness of many asymptomatic PHAs may have predisposed them to downplay the salience of HIV in their life and to refrain from thinking about far-off consequences. Many accepted their diagnosis as "part of my life" but refused to let it dominate and "put it to the back of my mind."

Another strategy was to accept the diagnosis without rancor and to develop a positive attitude in order to protect physical and mental health. Many participants mentioned the beneficial effects of successfully coping with an HIV diagnosis, and said that they felt stronger, more resilient, more thoughtful, and in some way a better person as a result of the process. Said Annie:

> I used to feel sorry for myself but then I sat down one day and I thought to myself what have I got to feel sorry for. I'm still in pretty good health. I've still got my son who loves me and I decided that I had to change my attitude towards a lot of things. ...I feel every day is a gift for me and like a bonus ... I love the simple things of life.

In addition to developing a positive attitude, Sandstrom (1990) also notes that some of the gay men he interviewed found that having AIDS gave them a sense of uniqueness and an expertise that was positively evaluated in certain social circles.

Despite little difference in psychological well being between PHAs and seronegatives, inspection of interview data revealed a marked difference in their feelings about the future. PHAs were much less optimistic than seronegatives about the future, which is not surprising given the deterioration in health and greatly curtailed life expectancy associated with AIDS. Other than addressing future concerns such as making wills or finding homes for their children, few PHAs felt able to make long-term plans (cf. Davies 1997). The lack of certainty about the future was voiced by many of the research subjects. Take, for example, the following interchange with Jim, a gay man who had been diagnosed a few months prior to his interview.

Jim: Now and again it really hits me.

GG: When are those sort of occasions?

Jim: It is when people start talking about the future. In fact I was just at the bank [with the] manager the other week there and he was like "You should really take out a long term savings plan and start doing this and that."

Few expressed fear of death itself but almost all were concerned about the process of dying; the asymptomatic participants feared the onset of severe symptoms and those with symptoms feared a painful and undignified death or physical dependence on others. Having a hopeless future orientation was also related to feelings of being robbed of a future. Parents, particularly mothers, expressed sadness at probably not being alive to witness their children's future life transitions.

However, many participants chose to focus upon positive aspects of their future and most felt relatively optimistic. Mick reported that his relationship with his father had become much closer as a result of his diagnosis, and Tony that it had prompted him to begin a drama course. Vicky and Heather, both living in a council housing estate (in US terms, a housing project) in Edinburgh said that HIV had widened their horizons and spoke proudly of their contributions at an AIDS conference they were sent to in Mexico. As Mary, an IDU who was looking forward to becoming a step-grandmother, told us, "I feel quite good and confident that I am going to be here for quite a while. As far as I am concerned I am not dying."

Key stages linking disease progression with psychosocial vulnerability were identified in the Scottish data. Acute psychological disturbance, notably anxiety, was reported in reaction to key stages in the illness careers of people with HIV, such as diagnosis, offer of treatment, onset of symptoms, and first hospitalization with an HIV-related illness.

Whilst a few people reported that their HIV diagnosis had not had a major impact upon them when they were initially informed,[10] many participants felt "out of control and hopeless" in the period just following diagnosis. Responses included bingeing on alcohol or street drugs, losing interest in appearance, and social withdrawal, and nine of the 66 said that they had tried to kill themselves at this time. Annie, an ex-IDU said she had attempted to drink herself to death when first diagnosed, to avoid AIDS appearing on her death certificate. Severe psychological distress in reaction to diagnosis can last for weeks, but by the time of interview the great majority of participants reported that they had "come to terms" with the diagnosis and that their lives had returned to a steady state.

The offer of treatment caused psychological distress among some participants. Of the 47 who were offered AZT,[11] ten experienced psychological trauma when offered it, interpreting the offer as a sign of progression. Development of symptoms was a constant source of distress even to those at an early stage of the illness. The more serious the symptom, the greater the accompanying stress, and hospitalization with an HIV-related symptom, particularly the first one, usually caused much anxiety. Said Lorrie, who was hospitalized with pneumonia, "I thought my number was up. I actually thought that was it. I was scared out of my mind." For many, hospitalization marked the first time they had really had to confront illness associated with HIV.

Confronting illness often caused distress, as most of the coping strategies of the asymptomatics involved classifying the disease into two stages: being 'well' and being 'ill'. Participants who clearly categorized themselves as being in the well stage while asymptomatic often felt forced by the onset of severe symptoms or hospitalization to recategorize themselves as ill, which was disruptive to their sense of self, at least for a time.

Notwithstanding the enormous variation in individuals' precise psychological trajectories following diagnosis, the findings clearly show that seropositive people are not very much more psychologically disturbed most of the time than seronegatives but that at particular times an HIV diagnosis can be an enormous burden. This crisis-point model we offer perhaps explains some of the contradictory findings in the literature, such as that while in the long term there seems to be little difference between seropositive people and seronegatives, there is a great deal of short-term stress associated with an HIV diagnosis.

The data suggest that the psychological strain of being seropositive is episodic. Thus, that a stronger relationship does not emerge between stage of illness, and psychological well being is likely to be related to the short-term nature of much HIV-related distress. In addition, much of the psychological distress that was reported by seropositive people was attributed to feelings or experience of stigma and ostracism rather than declining physical health. Among asymptomatics, this was often the cause of greater distress than coming to terms with having a chronic illness. The burden of disease progression and failing physical health was overshadowed by the social burden of HIV-related stigma.

However varied their psychological adjustment and coping styles may be, all PHAs have to confront the stigma associated with their illness – a stigma that, as we have seen, is associated with deviance, death, and danger. As Gary, a gay man, said: "The word 'AIDS' frightens a lot of people, not only those who have HIV but generally AIDS is one of those fearful words isn't it."

The word 'AIDS' terrifies most PHAs, at least when they first receive a diagnosis. The negative connotations of the term have a direct impact on their perception and management of social risk and may lead to self-devaluation and social withdrawal. This may reoccur during illness trajectory crisis points too, and to some degree affects life after diagnosis altogether: believing oneself to be diseased, dirty, and dangerous can alienate a PHA from his or her pre-diagnosis self and, consequently, from social relationships too. Psychosocial response to HIV and the various stages of psychological adaptation which follow are thus conjoined with adjustment to a new social identity – an HIV-identity which, in the eyes of many, is synonymous with a dangerous identity. It is this aspect of AIDS to which we now turn.

Reconstructing the self

Chronic illness and identity

In discussions of psychosocial adjustment to HIV infection, the impact that a positive test has on identity or self-concept has often been overlooked, despite the widely acknowledged connection between self-concept and psychological well being. Too often, measures of self-esteem or self-efficacy are deemed sufficient representations of self-concept and identity *per se* is not explored.

A number of authors have examined the relationship between illness and identity and the impact of chronic illness upon identity (e.g. Bury 1982; Charmaz 1983; Corbin and Strauss 1988). They show how the onset of chronic illness assaults not only the physical self but also a person's sense of identity and self-worth.

As with other chronic illnesses, HIV involves what Bury (1982: 167) refers to as "biographical disruption," i.e. a disruption of one's expected life trajectory. Bury (1991) identifies two types of 'meaning' in chronic illness which feed into this disruption. The first is the consequences of the illness for the individual and the manner in which symptoms and treatment regimes may disrupt everyday life. Much chronic illness, for example, enforces inactivity which, according to Herzlich and Pierret (1987: 178), "prevents individuals from 'playing their role', marginalizes them, and can even provoke a feeling of loss of identity. 'Who am I?' the sick person wonders. These questions sometimes reveal a feeling of total annihilation of the personality."

The second meaning identified by Bury is the significance of illness (the connotations and imagery of the illness) that may affect how people see themselves and how they think others see them. Mathieson and Stam (1995), who interviewed people with cancer, conceptualize this as "disrupted feelings of fit" (p. 293). Whilst disrupted feelings of fit may arise from disruption to regular routines due to a necessity to take medication etc., it essentially relates to a "confrontation with a new, alien, or changed social structure, in which the person's own role is changed too" (Jacobson-Widding 1983: 14, as cited in Mathieson and Stam 1995: 293). As one of their participants said "I suppose to my friends I'm Ruth with cancer, not just plain Ruth" (p. 294), and another reported a process whereby the illness is objectified and the person with cancer is seen "as a tumour, not as a person" (p. 296).

The disruption entailed underpins a renegotiation of identity that takes place between the chronically ill and their social milieu. This renegotiation involves major biography-altering facts, altered relationships, and a changed vision of the future, and the unpredictability inherent in this process ensures that uncertainty is a key aspect in the disruptive experience (Bury 1991). Uncertainty has indeed long been identified as a crucial issue for chronically ill persons (Conrad 1987; Glaser and Strauss 1968a; Wiener 1975; Royer 1998), particularly for those with HIV given the relative newness of the disease and its varied course (see Weitz 1989).

Most people are thus changed by illness, a change that is reflected in their social selves. Indeed, in extreme cases severe illness may signify social death. To quote a young mother interviewed in France in 1960 by Herzlich and Pierret (1987), "What is really so awful is that illness, I believe, really makes you very lonely. ...One is really out of the world. *When there is illness, one is and one stays, alone.* It's very hard to get help. ...It destroys what one would like to do, it isolates you" (p. 178; emphasis in original). A recent US study of the chronically ill also identifies social isolation as "the most devastating consequence" (Royer 1998: 26), as "social relationships are frequently disrupted and usually disintegrate under the stress of chronic illness and its management" (p. 65).

Today, many people with chronic illness reject the notion of social death and assert a right to participate fully in society.[12] Many dislike being categorized by their illnesses as 'the cancer patient' or 'the schizophrenic'. Because the immediate physical consequences of an HIV diagnosis are not generally as severe as with those of many other chronic illnesses, PHAs have played a key role in fighting for the rights of the chronically ill and they have helped to change attitudes towards chronic illness. However, the disruption that an HIV diagnosis entails is generally of sufficient severity to require 'biographical work' to recraft or reconstitute one's identity in the light of being HIV positive. As with all chronic illnesses, a process of legitimization and explanation is required whereby individuals try to find "explanations that make sense in terms of their life circumstances and biographies ... and re-establish credibility in the face of the assault on self-hood which is involved" (Bury 1991: 456).

Chronic illness requires strategic management to minimize the impact of illness on social interaction (Wiener 1975). Social risk, which everyone must manage, is compounded in the chronically ill by the stigmas associated with various chronic illnesses and the indeterminacy of their definition of self and of events. Writes Bury (1991: 454):

In responding to chronic illness, individuals constantly test the meanings attached to their altered situation against the reality of everyday experience. It is a situation of risk because individuals cannot be sure that their own developing perceptions and 'definition of the situation' will be shared by others, whether in the informal setting or in interactions with professional caregivers. Calls for help may turn out to produce unwanted dependence and calls for sympathy run the risk of rejection. Only the passage of time and trial and error can provide guidelines as to the nature of the risks involved in living with a particular condition, though a degree of unpredictability will always remain.

HIV and identity

The concept of identity, its upkeep and recreation, and the related role of story telling with reference to HIV were introduced in Chapter 2, and we have just discussed identity reconstruction in relation to chronic illness in general. Much that holds true in general holds true for PHAs too, although some difference is inevitable. Much of what little we know specifically about the concrete links between seropositivity and identity comes from studies carried out with bisexual and homosexual men. Sandstrom (1990) talks of the "drama of identity construction" (p. 271) of 19 gay men with AIDS-related diagnosis. He examines the process of identity construction in which "the illness is personalized and definitions of self are challenged, transformed, understood, and sustained" (p. 276). He notes also that identity management includes both defensive strategies to avoid potentially threatening or awkward social interactions and "forms of embracement ... to affirm an AIDS-related identity and to integrate it with other valued aspects of self" (p. 271). PHAs do the latter as they become more involved with AIDS support networks, and the HIV-positive community may thus play an important role in the construction of an HIV-positive identity (Roth and Nelson 1997).

As Lang (1991) explains, while many aspects of an individual's identity come into play in the coping process, the homosexual man's responses to an HIV or AIDS diagnosis "appear to be related to the prior social and psychological adjustment of the gay male to his sexual orientation" (p. 67). Those individuals who are "more constructive in this adjustment" (p. 67) – those who are neither closeted nor guilt-ridden – deal better with seropositivity than those who deny their sexual orientation or preference.

Lang's work suggests that coping strategies or styles and personal biography or identity constructions play key roles in mediating how people deal with HIV seropositivity. Indeed, after studying the personal narratives of seropositive homosexual young men, Borden found that "HIV seropositivity is likely to threaten existing interpretations of self, others, life experience, and anticipated future" (1991: 438). In other words, a positive HIV test may entail a need to revise one's life history, and this can be devastating.

A study conducted in France with 44 asymptomatic HIV-positive men infected homosexually or through haemophilia treatments found post-diagnosis identity reworking largely involved reinterpreting the past to strengthen a sense of self that pre-existed. The men reinforced "components of their identity which, prior to HIV infection, had already been built around haemophilia or homosexuality" (Carricaburu and Pierret 1995: 85). The men with haemophilia made no distinction between HIV and AIDS and they saw themselves as having AIDS even when, technically, they did not, as their notions of self had long been based around having an illness. The gay men, however, insisted on the distinction between HIV and AIDS and did not consider being HIV positive an illness state.

That identity is reformulated over the course of AIDS is well illustrated by Crossley (1997). She shows how a group of long-term HIV-positive individuals construct for themselves the identity of the 'healthy survivor', who is good, moral and responsible – the opposite of the unhealthy other who is different from the self. Unhealthy others are the weak-minded negative-thinking HIV-positive individuals, and the newly diagnosed, who the long-term survivors characterize as full of self-pity.

Studies suggest that newly seropositive people revise their life-stories to fit the test outcome, rethinking their worlds and their identities in relation to others in it. In regard to memory and narrative, Freeman has written that while "beginning leads to end, there is also a sense in which end leads to beginning, the outcome in question serving as the organizing principle around which the story is told" (1993: 20). In this way, a positive HIV test outcome[13] may lead a person to question previously accepted notions related to the self. A real sense of fragmentation may precede such revisionism.

For example, as noted in Chapter 2, seronegative women tell 'Monogamy Narratives' (Sobo 1993a, 1995b), in which their long-term partners are cast as loving, trustworthy, and sexually loyal. Yet, the women who participated in Ward's (Ward 1993b) research revised their stories after learning about their seropositive diagnoses, telling now of broken trust and partners, who did not really love them. 'Monogamy Narratives' turned to 'Betrayal Narratives' as the ramifications of the positive test were taken in and pictures of selves and others redeveloped in light of the newly discovered outcome.

Women who have internalized traditional role expectations must face their own imputed failure in fulfilling them upon testing positive. By dying of AIDS, they will not be able to fulfil their role as carers or nurturers, responsible for the well being of the next generation (Lawless *et al.* 1996). And the fact that they have been infected can be taken to mean that they were not doing a good mothering job before infection either. Their seropositive status leads to their symbolic association with prostitutes or women who retain ownership over their own sexuality rather than 'proper' women, who give that over to one man (Sacks 1996). HIV-positive women cannot fulfil role expectations – at least not in the traditional sense. And this can shatter previously taken-for-granted self-conceptions.

Despite HIV's ability to shatter identities, there is evidence suggesting that many people do not take social demotion lying down. Citing Bourdieu, Grove *et al.* (1997) argue that middle-class, monogamous women who do not inject drugs draw on "symbolic capital" to protect their moral statuses and identities. They distinguish themselves from members of so-called 'risk groups', actively "emphasizing the many nondeviant aspects of their lives" (p. 333) and eliciting sympathy for their plight as so-called 'innocent victims'. As noted in Chapter 2, however, this strategy perpetuates the retributional model and supports stigmatization of (other) PHAs.

While Grove *et al.* claim that mainstream women "experience a degree of latitude or control over their social fate that is not usually found among stigmatized individuals" (1997: 318), there is evidence to suggest that one actually need not be white, married, heterosexual, and a non-user of drugs to play such rhetorical games. From Hassin's study of the presentation of self among IDUs, we learn that "most of the users [she] met and spoke with rejected the 'junkie' caricature as applicable to themselves" (1994: 396). One HIV-positive IDU attempting to make her actions "understandable within the acceptable social norm" (p. 396) told Hassin stories demonstrating that she was a 'good' mother and an 'innocent victim' of AIDS. Likewise, the women mentioned above who told 'Betrayal Narratives' placed the responsibility for their HIV infection not on their own actions but on those of their mates. This despite the fact that, as poor women of colour, and generally unmarried, many others would cast them as inherently at risk.

Beside identity *per se*, the point in the life course, and the point in the course of the illness at which a positive diagnosis is made may affect the manner in which one reinterprets the events of one's life and reinvents the self. So may the degree to which HIV threatens life plans and daily routines. Indeed, a loss of self-anchoring, self-unifying everyday aspects of life might lead some HIV-positive people to engage more intensely in negotiations related to identity. Concentrated engagement with such issues may be associated with crisis points, such as when cell counts fall below a certain point, or a hospital admission, or certain social situations, for example those in which stigma leads to bias. The stigma of AIDS can lead PHAs to experience intense social and moral confusion (Earl *et al.* 1991–92).

Dangerous identities, tainted selves

Perceiving oneself as having a tainted identity or of being somehow different is the hallmark of possessing a stigma, as Goffman originally defined it (1963). Socio-cultural norms underlie stigma and members of a society who are stigmatized internalize socio-cultural attitudes towards them – attitudes expressed in discrimination (such as dismissal from employment or rejection by social contacts). They thus feel themselves to be tainted as well as despised. In this manner stigma becomes a two way process ensuing between the stigmatized individual and society.[14]

We now examine the elements of dangerousness that PHAs may be associated with and internalize, paying special attention to PHAs own perceptions regarding the symbolic basis of the stigmatization. Although we focus below (as above) on the Scottish data, there were numerous similar reports from all our study sites.

Dirty Lepers

A number of people in the Scottish sample compared being seropositive to feeling "like a leper," or "as if I had the plague." Cathy, a heterosexual, said she felt like a leper when she had her tooth removed in a general hospital because she was put in a side ward, away from other patients; further, "The nurses stayed away from me. They wouldn't even touch my clothes unless they had some gloves on." Mick told of his boyfriend's fear of touching him, saying, "It bothers me. He stays overnight and he sleeps on the same bed but there is no cuddling or anything. I feel like a leper at times."

Many PHAs in the Scottish sample reported knowing at least one person who did not want to socialize with them anymore because of their HIV status, and others had seen this happen to other PHAs. For example, Annie, an ex-IDU, said:

> Anybody that found out I had the virus I got rejected. People just didn't want to know, people stopped coming to my house and when they saw

> me coming along the street they would cross the road. ...Even my so-called best pal, she took her two kiddies' hands and walked across the street ... I felt a right outcast.

Participants also reported overhearing comments from people unaware of their positive serostatus or reading things in newspaper articles that made them feel tainted or part of a shunned group. Thomas, who was living in a house for recovering alcoholics, was sitting in the common room shortly after his diagnosis. He had not disclosed his serostatus to the other residents. He said, "One guy was reading in the paper and he turned round and said to me, 'See all them with AIDS they should be rounded up and put them on an island and sink it'." Likewise Sheila went to visit a friend soon after her diagnosis only to hear the friend's mother say, not knowing Sheila's status, that she would not have a positive person in her house.

An HIV-positive person's identity is tainted to the extent that the person with HIV believes him- or herself dirty or perceives that others will think this to be so. James responded to his diagnosis by "washing everything. I wash my hands all the time." Marie, an IDU, said she would not let anyone touch her for months after her diagnosis. The dirtiness associated with HIV is particularly well illustrated in the following conversation with Betty, an IDU:

Betty: I felt dirty and unclean for a long time.

GG: Why was that do you think?

Betty: Because of the way this disease came about, know what I mean, it was poofs [gays] and then it was sex so it had a dirty image, know what I mean to it. And then it was all gays and it was their fault and then it was drug addicts. It's always had a stigma and been a dirty disease, know what I mean, so you do feel people go 'Ooh' and [all] that. People don't go 'Ooh' if you've got cancer or leukemia, know what I mean. It was the way it was brought about I think.

Despite having been diagnosed for five years Betty had still not told her 12-year old son because "he might feel he's dirty." Likewise, Cathy, infected heterosexually, had not told her 18-year old son; if he knew "he'd go crazy because he thinks only dirty people get it."

The infectious identity

A great deal of stigma is attached to having any infectious disease, whether HIV or contagious dermatitis. People with flu or a cold are generally kept at arm's length, and we encourage those with large numbers of visible lesions, as with chickenpox, to isolate themselves.

Although routes of HIV transmission are very limited, people's fear of transmission, as noted in Chapter 2, is large. Many PHAs in our studies said that even close relatives were frightened of contagion. John reported, "For a couple of days my sister-in-law was all on edge when I stayed at their house. It was like your own knife and fork and plate." Janice said that her boyfriend's brother "takes his own plates and cups when he visits his mother," in order to avoid using those that may have been previously used and contaminated by Janice.

Sometimes, perception related to contagion led to apparently unnecessary isolation. Said Heather of her hospitalization for childbirth, "They moved my bed out of the ward away up the back, paper sheets honest to God. When they came into my room they had masks on and that they were like spacemen. I was not allowed to use the same toilet as the others." As Mick put it, "There's people out there that think if they look at you they're going to get it."

Other times, isolation was self-imposed, due to stigma internalization. Ian explained, "My neighbour recently had a baby and when she came back from the hospital she must have wondered – I just didn't want to touch the baby." Sometimes, PHAs see this type of response as irrational even as they do it: Morag said about her niece, "If I'm drinking tea I wouldn't let her drink out the same cup as me even though she couldn't catch it from that."

All participants were aware of the public opprobrium directed at anyone who puts others at risk of contagion. Some reasoned that public disapproval was misplaced and that tagging or quarantining people with HIV would be "just a horrible infringement of human rights." Others, however, shared the public's fear and hatred of people with HIV who put others at risk.

During the study a national news story came out about a man with haemophilia who had supposedly knowingly infected at least four women with HIV. A participant with haemophilia commented, "The guy is a bit of a dot really. Personally I think he should be charged with attempted murder." Another said, "If you're hunting for women and you're HIV positive you should be tagged." The great majority expressed strong disapproval of any PHA who had unprotected sex with an untested or seronegative partner without disclosing to them first – even those who had done so themselves. In addition, many said it was unethical for PHAs to have a child (including one mother who had become pregnant and given birth after her diagnosis).

By voicing such positions, HIV-positive people actively cast themselves as moral beings who share the convictions of the mainstream. However, they also acknowledge the understanding that some PHAs are, indeed, morally corrupt and dangerous beings. If internalized, whether wholly or in part, this type of knowledge can damage one's self-worth.

Many participants felt dangerous not only because of the possibility of infecting others but also because their stigma itself was contagious. Thomas said his major concern was for his partner: he worried about how "people would treat her being with somebody like me." Vanessa had similar concern for her partner, Harold; she said, "I don't want people turning 'round and saying like 'You don't want to go near that [Harold] he has probably got AIDS or something because his bird [girlfriend] has got it'."

Many PHAs with young children worried that their children would suffer a courtesy stigma if their diagnoses become widely known, and concern also was expressed for parents. As Morag said, "If any of us [kids] died it would cause [my parents] hurt but I'm causing them additional hurt, dying of this, dying of AIDS."

AIDS = death

Another factor fueling the outsider status of PHAs is that they have a terminal illness for which no cure or vaccine as yet exists; although they may appear healthy and feel healthy, and despite new breakthroughs in managing the disease, PHAs are still seen as dying. There is a wide literature on the stigma accompanying terminal illness (e.g. Sontag 1991) and many PHAs are assumed near death, even though many live for years after diagnosis. Despite its ubiquity, death has very negative connotations in US and UK culture and PHAs are linked with danger due to their imputed link with death.

Robbie told us that when he first entered prison after being diagnosed, there was a flat in Hall A for people with HIV that was nicknamed "death row." Robert, also a prisoner, said of his reputation, "There were lots of rumours but I was healthy and they thought an AIDS victim was like a skeleton." The expression 'death sentence' was commonly used to describe AIDS: "When they first told me I had the virus I thought it was a death sentence," Annie told us. And, in a macabre turn of events reported by Vanessa, "When my dad found out he told people that I had died of AIDS and that. There was even people coming up to my brother and asking when the funeral was."

Other illnesses

Given the danger associated with AIDS, it was common for people to 'cover' by telling, or implying to others, that they were suffering from a less discrediting disease. Cover diseases tend to be those which share some of the symptoms of the different stages of HIV infection, such as Chronic Fatigue Syndrome (historically called Myalgic Encephalomyelitis or ME in the UK), which is associated with generalized fatigue and malaise. Various forms of cancer were also used as cover diseases as they may be associated with weight loss, hospitalization and death.

David told us of his employer, "I would rather he thought I had ME than HIV because there is a greater stigma attached to HIV." Speaking of her parents, Morag said, "I think they will get to know eventually but even if I am sick I will tell them it is cancer. Even if I die I still don't want them to know about it." Derek told his ten-year old son and most of his close friends that he has lung cancer. Janice told people she has epilepsy; Mark told them he has Hepatitis B. Some use still other diseases as their covers.

Covering HIV-related illness by naming another disease was often felt to be necessary to avoid AIDS's stigma while at the same time laying a claim to being ill. The rationale for this is well illustrated by Vanessa, who had been asked to present for a repeat cervical smear as the first one had produced ambivalent results. She said:

> I was in the clinic and that and the nurse like was saying to me before I went in to see the doctor, she was saying like, "Don't worry, it does not mean to say that you have got cancer. They just want to do a repeat test." I says, "Look I am HIV, if I have got cancer it is more socially acceptable to have cancer than HIV so I am not worried about it." I says, "If I have got cancer at least I can turn round and say to people well I'm dying of cancer" and they will accept that. If you turn round and say you are HIV they run away from you.

HIV as 'The Other'

We have previously noted that the stigma literature argues that people make distinctions and barriers between the 'healthy self' and the 'unhealthy other' (e.g. Crawford 1994). This distinction can be made for a society, in an us-them equation, or it can be made for or within an individual, who has good and bad components, or has some dimensions that s/he simply will not own. In some people the stigmatized other is conceptualized as essentially different from the normal self. Still, sometimes the stigma overshadows and even overwhelms the person underneath.

As Gina explained, "Sometimes I'd like to tell other people but I know I can't because of the stigma and everything." Peter simply said, "I want people to think of me as me and not as the guy with HIV." Annie told us, "People still sort of draw back and you see them talking behind your back and that. I passed people one day just round the corner. I had gone out to post a letter and I heard as clear as anything, 'That's her that's got AIDS'."

The sense of otherness that disclosing one's serostatus could entail was reinforced by participants' high awareness of AIDS's association with already-stigmatized groups – for example with, as one woman called them, "bloody perverts and drug addicts." Said Patrick, a man with haemophilia, "Articles started to appear in all the newspapers. Basically it was all related to drug users, homosexuals and that sort of thing. I did not really want to be in that category." Gina, who did not use drugs and was neither promiscuous nor gay, said "I just hate the stigma people have towards it. You must be a junkie or you must be sleeping with absolutely everyone or you're gay. People don't seem to think you can get it by your partner." Imputed blame caused further problems for some participants. Many reported that some family and friends had blamed them for becoming infected and felt it would have been avoidable had they lived their lives differently. Similar opinions were voiced by the New Mexican and North-East England samples in regard to this and all of the above issues.

Degrees of danger

Deviance and danger are relative concepts. As Becker (1963) shows in his classic work *Outsiders*, what is deviant for one person in one place and time may be classified as benign for another person or the same person at a different place or time. For example, in the early twentieth century, unmarried mothers were often classified as mentally ill and institutionalized, whereas today one in three children in Britain is born outside wedlock. In most offices, cinemas and an increasing number of restaurants in England smoking is prohibited, whereas in parts of Spain cigars are distributed to – and expected to be smoked by – all adult wedding guests. Obesity, seen as decadent in the UK and USA, is highly regarded in many poorer societies as evidence of affluence (*cf.* Sobo 1993b).

The degree to which an act or illness is regarded as deviant depends on who commits the act or who has the illness and who has been harmed or threatened by it. As Sutherland (1940) shows in his analysis of white-collar crime, crimes committed by corporations are usually prosecuted as civil cases whereas the same crimes are usually treated as criminal offences when committed by individuals. Likewise, a person with a mental illness who is charged with assault may be in one context directed to mental health services, and in another sent to prison.

To quote Becker, "Deviance is not a quality that lies in behaviour itself, but in the interaction between the person who commits an act and those who respond to it" (1963: 14). The danger associated with being HIV positive is defined in the same manner, that is, by the interaction between the person who has the illness and the response of the self and wider society. In this way, the danger that HIV represents and the degree to which it shatters identity varies for each person with HIV.

As noted, the experiences and feelings described by members of the Scottish sample and reported above also were described at the other sites. However, individually, PHAs have such experiences, feelings, or opinions to different degrees or not at all. Individual differences seem to be at least partly related to the perceived fit between the individual in question and the stereotypic PHA. While we did not recognize any significant US-UK differences except perhaps in turns of phrase, we did document some differences according to whether participants were male or female, their self-reported mode of infection, and sexual preference. These differences are discussed in Chapter 11.

Another factor affecting one's perceived fit with the stereotypic HIV-positive person is one's position on the rural-urban or parochial-cosmopolitan continuum, but for this, as for class and race or ethnicity, we did not have a wide enough sampling net to observe such differences in our samples. However, as Peter Keogh has suggested (personal communication, 1996[15]), the types of self-reports and rhetoric that we describe may be uncommon among many urban gay men who belong to supportive communities or sex-positive networks. The politics of blame may run differently for, or simply be of no interest to, such men. When a positive HIV test is seen to reflect the immorality of homophobic sociopolitical and medical systems, or as purely a matter of chance, people are less likely to report feelings like those discussed above. Nor will they need to engage in negotiations such as those we describe in Chapters 6–10.

Whatever one's perceived degree of danger – however one internalizes the stigmatization associated with AIDS – the PHA always must deal with the question of self-disclosure, or of 'telling'. The next chapter examines the issues PHAs confront when deciding whether or not (and how much) to expose their positive status. With the next chapter, then, we begin to look in more depth at the strategies and techniques by which PHAs in our studies navigated the HIV-specific landscape of social risk.

Notes

1 This may change as symptoms worsen and access to certain AIDS services becomes necessary.

2 We also cannot know whether any of the few people who contacted us directly after having heard about the studies rather than having been put in contact with us by AIDS service organizations' gatekeepers (four people in England, two people in Scotland, and no people in the USA) were actually seropositive, as we did not demand test results of them nor did we corroborate their claims by looking into their medical records. We relied only on self-reported serostatus and health claims. Even those referred directly by gatekeepers may have been seronegative people 'working the system' to their benefit (*cf.* Huby 1999). However, the testimony of each participant did ring true, and the insider knowledge demonstrated provided more than enough evidence to convince us that each and every participant was indeed seropositive.

3 Participants in an Australian study saw negative test results as useful in sexual negotiations; men in particular often said that once they had had an HIV test they did not need to continue with using condoms" (Lupton *et al.* 1995).

4 With publisher permission, this section on adjusting to a positive test updates and expands upon Chapter 4 in Sobo (1995b).

5 The little we have read about this in relation to men as fathers has been anecdotal; research related to pediatric AIDS has ignored the male role.

6 Barbara Limandri uses the word "colonizing" to describe the latter process, in which people with similar conditions seek one another out (1989: 77).

7 Much of this section is based on Green, Platt, Eley, and Green (1996).

8 While methodological details were provided in the preceding chapter, for full details regarding the research see (Green *et al.* 1996).

9 Even now, new treatment options are only available to a select few and a lack of access may make psychological health worse for those who know they are or who perceive themselves to be cut off from them.

10 The people with haemophilia who were tested in the early to mid-1980s, for example, often did not understand the full implications of the diagnosis and considered it to be "just another thing," rather like Hepatitis B, which many haemophiliacs get as a result of their use of blood products.

11 AZT, the common term for Zidovudine, was the drug most commonly prescribed to slow down the rate of progression during the fieldwork period.

12 The social movement that promotes the social participation of disabled people is based on a model that views disability within the social contexts constructed by and for the dominant group of non-disabled people (Oliver 1990). In this model, the problem lies in the exclusion of impaired people from social institutions, and disability can best be overcome by society learning to adapt to the diverse nature and abilities of its citizens.

13 The experience of HIV-related sicknesses, offer of treatment, etc., may serve as a reminder and index of one's positive test outcome and so may result in the same processes to be described in the text here.

14 This is not to say that those with known stigmatizing conditions who do not accept socio-cultural norms and who do not internalize society's negative judgment of themselves are unaffected by stigma. They are still at risk of stigmatization from others. Furthermore, the degree to which any individual living in a given society can reject socio-cultural norms is probably small; even if these norms are somewhat rejected, certain aspects of them will be accepted and so certain aspects of stigma will be internalized.

15 This comment was in response to a seminar paper presented by Sobo on February 29, 1996, as part of the Bloomsbury Medical Anthropology Seminar Series at University College London. The paper was titled, 'Concealing Positive HIV Serostatus From Sexual Partners: The Seropositive Person's Point of View'.

Chapter 6

Telling

The self-disclosure challenge

Across all sites, most seropositive participants were asymptomatic and healthy and only a very few looked seriously ill.[1] They told us that they mostly chose to try to pass as seronegative ('normal') by keeping their serostatus to themselves.

According to Goffman's conceptualization of stigma in relation to identity, by omitting accurate serostatus information from their public identity claims, these participants assumed a 'discreditable' identity. By definition, the concept implies secrecy and shame.

While it is true that those who conceal a stigma may feel as if they keep a shameful secret that, if exposed, would be discrediting, the automatic assumption of concealment and shame when stigma is not openly self-applied is unwarranted. The PHA who has not internalized the cultural connotations of AIDS might not see him- or herself as discreditable at all. As shown in Chapter 5, many asymptomatic people with HIV see themselves as 'not sick' and as definitely not having AIDS, although as Jamie (England) said, much of the public "can't make that distinction [between HIV and AIDS] in their minds."

Further, putting one's HIV serostatus out of awareness much of the time or not invoking it as an essential aspect of identity is not necessarily the same as purposefully concealing it or denying it. Being selective about who knows about it may not hinge on having a personal belief that it is discrediting. It does, however, entail an understanding that many others who might judge them do feel it is discrediting.

Due largely to concerns regarding such judging others, the majority of participants sustained non-HIV-linked public identities. But the same was not so within
their personal social networks. In the Scottish sample, for example, all but one
person interviewed had told at least one person in their social network that they
were HIV positive. On average respondents had told three-quarters of their close
social contacts.[2]

This chapter examines why people feel the need to disclose to members of their
social networks, and how they decide whom to tell. The next chapter focuses upon
the dangers that discourage disclosure. Both chapters focus on the process of risk
assessment related to HIV self-disclosure and highlight the cultural ideals and models
that underlie many disclosure decisions. While later chapters examine disclosure
among members of specific samples to specific subsets of social relations (health
care workers in Scotland and sexual partners in England and New Mexico), this
and the next chapter take a broad approach that is not site-specific. We examine a
diverse array of examples of telling in an effort to outline the general issues that
came up in the narratives of disclosure decision-making that we collected.

At each site, locally meaningful norms, mores, and modes of expression coloured
the specific stories we were told. This surface variation and its context-specific
importance notwithstanding, the same general ideals and models were mentioned
over and over by participants at each site when they talked about self-disclosure.
The similarities support claims that our Scottish, English, and US PHAs participate
jointly in an at least somewhat-shared cultural system (i.e. Western culture). They
also suggest that there may be some universal aspects of the experience of living
with HIV or AIDS. However, the degree to which the aspects we have identified
are present or taken note of in any society may differ according to the degree to
which Western influences are felt (and Western treatment opportunities available).

The initial factors participants introduced when talking about telling were the
same as have previously been reported (e.g. Hays *et al.* 1993). The person disclosed
to – the disclosee – could reject or abandon the self-discloser; s/he might even tell
others of the discloser's condition. Moreover, self-disclosure can involve revealing
damning (culturally unacceptable) information about one's conjugal relations (or
one's drug use patterns) and this can be degrading as well as possibly leading
to negative consequences such as loss of a primary partner or physical attack. It
also can entail having to face facts about oneself (or one's partner, and one's
relationship) that were more comfortable left unacknowledged and unincorporated
into one's identity.

Findings from all three sites indicate that basic mainstream cultural models were
at the root of these perceived risks and of self-disclosure decisions. Higher-order
models about morality and goodness came into play as people justified their self-

disclosure decisions as 'right' or moral. More specific models – models for friend-ship, familial, and conjugal relations – underwrote, to a large degree, the ways that people talked about the specific 'dos and don'ts' of self-disclosure.

For example, certain standards of conduct applied with friends, relatives, and lovers that did not apply with others. In explaining self-disclosure decisions related to friends, relatives, and lovers, participants commonly drew on models for informa-tion sharing linked to friendship, kinship, and conjugal ideals. In particular, they brought up understandings about the importance of sharing potentially damaging personal or private information for building and maintaining such relationships. Models for information sharing and the conjugal, kinship, and friendship models they were linked to played a very important role in self-disclosure decision-making among our participants, providing a basis for certain key aspects of risk evaluation.

Use of these models is troubled by the contradictory notion that trust, which ideally is a stable part of friendship, kinship, or conjugality, actually is an unstable element. Even one's most trusted confidants may betray through an unwanted response to disclosure, or by sharing the confidence with others. A close friend, for example, who calmly accepts a PHA's disclosure embodies a space of safety, but the same friend may become dangerous if the relationship sours.

Testing the waters

Self-disclosure decision-making generally happens over time. In a study of self-disclosure of a number of stigmatizing conditions including HIV seropositivity, Limandri (1989) found that self-disclosers generally "conceal for awhile, disclose, then retract back into concealment" (p. 73), searching for signs that full revelation will not result in rejection. If such signs are forthcoming, disclosure then can be "invitational" (the self-discloser provides clues, inviting the disclosee to make inquiries), or "reciprocal" (in which the disclosee reciprocates with some kind of self-disclosure in return).[3]

Data from any of our three sites contain numerous examples of both disclosure styles; in this section we quote the men interviewed in North-East England, who were specifically asked about self-disclosure strategies. Timothy said, "I think what I do subconsciously is to go through some kind of testing routine with people." Matthew stated frankly, "I like testing people to see how they can cope with different bits of information and seeing whether they are worthy or not."

Some disclosures were specifically reciprocal or invitational. Frank's story of a reciprocal disclosure shows how revelations of HIV serostatus also can entail other disclosures:

[My friend] confided and he told me that ... he used to be em a heroin addict and so I figured well it's took him all his time to tell me that ... I could tell by the way he was speaking he really needed someone to confide in. He said, "You haven't got any secrets like that have you?" So I figured well it might make him feel a little bit better if I told him about myself so I did. And I told him about my sexuality and all that shit.

When people spend time searching for positive or negative signs they are making an analysis of the risk landscape. Just as the poker player looks at the cards in his or her hand as well as those exposed on the table and considers what might be left in the pack when making a decision about whether or not to raise the stakes or fold, so the person with HIV has a sense of assessing the landscape to decide whether or not to disclose their HIV status to individual contacts. And just like the poker player, the PHA often asks, "What's in this for me?"

For example, when Malcolm was diagnosed, he was at university. He explained, very rationally, the risk calculations he went through in deciding whether to tell his instructors:

The first thing I sort of weighed up was, er, what do I stand to gain and what do I stand to lose by disclosure and, for example, in the case of lecturers [in the USA, instructors or professors] it was a case of I cannot predict how my health will go during the course. ...[I] do good quality work and don't want my grades to suffer in the event of a late submission because I was too ill or too tired, em, so I thought about it and I thought about the boundaries of confidentiality that lecturers will be bound to and I thought well I can nail their arses to the wall if they do anything that compromises me in any way whatsoever so I'll tell them because then they will also be aware of my circumstances and sort of it could benefit me with regard to my degree. So it was a case of what can I get out of it and how safe am I in disclosing to them, who else will they disclose to and if they disclose what can I do.

So in some cases, determining whether to disclose is rather cut and dried and costs and benefits are carefully considered.[4] However, just as the poker player has to judge the cards in his or her hand and on the table, s/he also has to interpret signs from the other players (e.g. a cough, a raised eyebrow, a laugh) to determine whether they are holding good hands or bluffing. This human element complicates calculations. Judging others involves intuition, emotion and feeling, all of which may wax and wane according to the risk landscape, the composition of which – and the

PHA's perception of which – constantly fluctuates. Thus, most disclosure decisions were not retold as if so overtly calculating; even when economic language was used, the riskiness of the endeavour was generally expressed in a visceral fashion, and for most, the sense of risk described or anticipated ran high.

For instance, Jamie, rehearsing for his interviewer the disclosure he was planning to make to a new partner, imagined, "I'd say, 'Well look there's something you've got to know about, em you're not going to like what you hear but I feel that I've got to tell you ... em I'm HIV positive' – and then I'd just walk out of the room and light up sort of like 700 fags [cigarettes] all in one go! [laughs]"

Risk can lead to fear and dread such as that which Jamie's statement about nervous smoking (and his assumption, "you're not going to like what you hear") manifests, but it also can be exciting. Like placing a bet on the horses, which entails the promise of a windfall as well as of utter defeat, the risk of disclosing also can entail an arousing thrill. Further, seropositivity is not a nice thing, and sometimes participants spoke of enjoying the rise it created in others. For example, Malcolm said:

> If I feel comfortable somehow from some connection between that person then I can say it and get away with it. 'Cos it is a bit like "Can I get away with it today?" kind of thing and I am sure there is an element of enjoyment in it that I get out of the shock factor as well, which is pretty sad.

Malcolm builds himself up by demonstrating that he is moral enough to know to chastise himself for enjoying shocking others; moreover, he demonstrates a belief in the notion that closer relationships are supposed to be more unconditional (a notion to which we later return). At the same time, he conveys through his talk of "getting away with it" the sense of risk that disclosure entails. And he displays ambivalence about his need for others and his need for self-protection. For in effect he says that while he is vulnerable to rejection he will maintain the power to reject others first, by shocking them with his disclosure, and the shock he gives them will be more damaging to them than any shock or rejection they in turn might deliver.

Who has a need to know?

Self-disclosure risk assessments, whether carefully considered or relatively sponta-neous, were often conceptualized by PHAs at all three sites as according with a process of identifying those who 'need to know'. David from Scotland explained,

"I think you have to sit and think 'Well who do I need to know and why do I need them to know? What good is it going to do me and what good is it going to do them?'"

Participants' definitions of those who needed to know often did not include those who were, technically speaking, most at risk of HIV transmission, such as casual sexual partners with whom risky behaviours were practised. Although risk for infection did figure, the need to know was related first and foremost to the possible social risks of disclosure. If it was deemed more risky, socially, to conceal one's serostatus from a given person, then that individual needed to know. The phrase 'need to know' – used a myriad of times by participants from all sites – reflects, however indirectly, the notion that information is a commodity, the exchange of which can lead to profits and losses that will have direct ramifications for self-protection.

Generally, a person's need to know hinged on the goals that the PHA held for the relationship with the person in question. Relationships were plotted on a continuum of closeness, with strangers at the end farthest from the PHA and sexual partners and kin with whom the PHA desired good relations at the near end.[5] The closer a person was seen to be, the more important self-disclosure became.

The respectable, moral self

In addition to and as part of the 'need to know' concept (and the social distance or closeness it entailed), narratives of disclosure decision-making centred on moral imperatives.[6] In Chapter 2, we argued that most narratives are teleological and concerned with "the good;" most talk of events or actions contrives them as part of a movement toward certain culturally-relative presupposed – and moral – ends (MacIntyre 1985). Rymes (1995), who has examined the construction of moral agency in the narratives of US high-school drop-outs, goes so far as to say that in telling stories people are "forced to articulate a moral orientation" (p. 499).

A moral orientation need not necessarily implicate good and evil as such. MacIntyre's "the good" (1985) might be better described as a model of how the world is, or how the world and the actors in it *should* be. Further, the moral orientation reported by the speaker need not be the one s/he actually holds but may rather be the one s/he thinks that the listener believes in – especially when the speaker accords him- or herself less authority than the listener.

For example, youths may tell a teacher that drug use is bad because that is what they know the teacher would prefer to hear; it benefits them to take that stance with the teacher. Further, what is bad here and now might be good in another context; youths might see drug use as bad in school or church but fine at home amongst friends. They might see drug use as good for themselves, but bad for a younger age group. And if they do not use drugs but know the teacher does, they may say drug use is fine, just to be polite.

While people are, as Rymes argues, "actively narrating themselves relative to a moral ideal of what it is to be a good person" (1995: 498), people do play, and people do deceive one another as well as acting as co-conspirators in upholding other's claims. Even in the most intimate conversations people must manage the ways that others see them and this necessarily affects the moral ideals that speakers appeal to.

The participants in this research certainly held paradigmatic cultural models of how the world should be, as do we all. As later examples will show, in telling their stories, they constructed their actions, or their responses to their actions, or the actions or words of others, as moral or as culturally correct.[7] Cultural models for sex, romance, and gender relations as well as models for kinship and friendship often came into play as participants compared their own AIDS-related actions and those of others to those recommended by the community with which they identified.[8]

Before providing examples, it bears noting that narrative self-creations are contingent and can be fleeting. They can change shape with one narrative turn. They may both contribute to and reflect the constantly changing landscape of risk. The creative dimension of narrative, which is constantly generating versions of self, albeit shifting ones, springs from its inter-subjective nature. That is, it has to do with the fact that people talk about themselves to others, imagined or real, rather than in complete social vacuums. And the reactions of others (again, imagined or real) can have profound effects on the shape that one's version of self takes over the course of a monologue or conversation.

All this needs bearing in mind when reviewing the self-reports we present as evidence of our findings. For the self-reports are not simply statements about events or feelings, they are simultaneously claims to, and active efforts at, the construction of self as good, moral, and upstanding. This is very important in light of the negative stigma that PHAs may be fighting.

Constructing the moral self through telling

To protect others

Each participant ascribed a high 'need to know' to people they were close to and felt to be at risk of HIV transmission by virtue of their relationship to him or her. Closer relationships by cultural definition entail trust, which the participants felt leads many to let their HIV guard down. So, people with closer relations to a PHA were seen by that PHA as in need of extra protection – as having a big need to know.

With very few exceptions, participants expressed an obligation to disclose to long-term regular sexual partners so that those partners might make informed decisions regarding whether to have sex with them and, sometimes more importantly, to diffuse potential trouble should these partners become infected. Billy, a Scottish ex-IDU, who had infected a former girlfriend prior to his own diagnosis, explained, "I think you have a duty to tell a girl even though a lot of guys would just say 'Oh pull on a condom and carry on'. I still think you have a duty because there is evidence that a condom can burst you know." By invoking the notion of duty and showing himself as more careful and caring than "a lot of guys" Billy stakes a strong claim to his own moral personhood.

Billy also demonstrated knowledge about the risks entailed even in safer sex. Likewise, a member of the English sample said:

> If we were a hundred per cent sure about the routes of transmission and we were totally aware that every single thing that we had done at that particular moment was safe with that person then I could argue that there is no need for disclosure but I don't think that we are in a position scientifically to be able to say that at the moment.

Disclosure to sexual partners is discussed in more detail in Chapters 9 and 10; here we would highlight the strategic deployment of the understanding that, especially in the face of scientific uncertainty, disclosing is a logically defensible moral imperative in sexual situations that entail risks for partners.[9] Participants made sure interviewers knew that they shared this understanding and so were 'good' people.

Because of uncertainty about transmission modes, some felt it was their duty to inform housemates, particularly in circumstances where sharing toothbrushes or razors was common. Likewise, some that felt that their occupations might place others at risk and so felt they had a duty to stop working or change jobs. For example, Lorrie (Scotland) elected to give up his job as an assistant chef in case he cut himself when chopping food.

It also was often seen as necessary to inform health professionals who were or might be at risk during the course of routine health care. A Scottish participant "told the dentist because it was an extraction and I knew there was going to be blood and that." He and others acted to safeguard their health-care providers from the risk of transmission, and in talking about their actions they demonstrated that they were good people despite what might have been said about them as PHAs (for more on morality and identity among PHAs, see Chapter 10; medical experiences *per se* are discussed in Chapter 8).

Many participants felt a need to tell all friends with children. Marie, a Scottish IDU, said, "I think my friends that have got young children should know." Others from Scotland explained: "People that I tell like for the simple reason as like my friend has got wains [small children] and that;" and "I wouldn't play with anyone's kids unless they knew." Ian told a female friend because "she had just got a new baby and that;" Morag told a couple she knew "because they had kids."

The compulsion to disclose where children are concerned is perhaps best illustrated in a story told by Gina, a Scottish participant studying for qualifications to work in a nursery. She enjoyed her course but had problems related to a form her supervisor had to fill in to comply with the Children's Act to confirm "that this person is fit to look after children." Neither HIV nor AIDS were specifically mentioned on the form, but her supervisor, to whom she had disclosed, was unsure whether to sign it.

> As far as my supervisor is concerned I am fit. But it's just that for some reason if it got out that I was HIV positive well you can imagine how parents would feel. You know they'd be terrified and I can understand. ...So he's got to see various people about that before he actually signs the forms to keep himself in the right and also to keep me in the right.

Despite widespread knowledge that risk resulting from interacting socially with children is no more than theoretical, participants in Scotland felt that children should be protected from them, or at least that children's parents should be informed so that they could decide whether or not the PHA was a danger to their child. That participants knew they were not actually a physical danger to children[10] is illustrated in the following interchange:

John: I did not want them thinking I had been in their house with this thing among kids.

GG: But you knew that you weren't a danger for the kids?

John: Aye, but did they know. I wanted them to know to be aware that I had the virus.

For most, the need to disclose to protect children seemed to hinge on a self-perceived identity as dangerous. Timothy (England) said, "It got to a point where I no longer saw myself as anything other than a virus." Seropositivity, at certain times or in certain contexts, tainted the participants; it made them unsuitable companions for children, or at least it made them people whom a child's parents may think this about. Some therefore reasoned that it was safer to tell parents of children they mixed with than to risk the potential danger of a parent finding out later and accusing them of endangering their child. In addition, avoiding interaction with children helped bolster for many the sense that they were good, moral people: they were 'doing the right thing' – striving to safeguard others, and honouring parents' rights over deciding what's best for their own children.

Whilst children were thus seen as high-risk contacts best avoided by many PHAs in our studies, for others – particularly parents – they were an invaluable source of support and represented safety. In the USA, Janie asserted that "Children are more supportive than I feel others would be. ...Their minds are open to learn and understand." This was echoed by members of the focus group she was part of, who also noted that children's attitudes towards them served as examples to others. Meg said that "children do help the partner to develop, 'cos they're so honest and they still love you. It helps that partner to see that. 'The child loves her and I should too.' Or, 'Kids aren't scared, why should I be?'" Maria pointed out, "That child just loves you, just unconditionally ... no matter how sick or how bad you look. That child will always love you, and that also gives a partner that other perspective. ...Even my mother – my son has given my mom strength in learning to love me all over again."

Attitudes of PHAs towards children make manifest the multi-layered and shifting notions of safety and danger that are part of each PHAs landscape of risk. Interaction with children is dangerous (socially risky) because others may perceive PHAs as a danger to them. Yet children are also seen as innocent, open, honest and a source of unconditional love and safety or sanctuary for PHAs. Their love for and acceptance of PHAs is used by participants to demonstrate that PHAs are not immoral monsters but rather good people, as worthy of love as those without antibodies to HIV.

Assertion of identity

A willingness to protect others, even though it may entail risks to oneself (via self-disclosure), was key in the moral identity that many participants constructed for themselves in the interview context. But one's identity itself also was seen, by many, as in need of safeguarding. Many felt that disclosing helped them avoid 'living a lie'.

Always having to live as if seronegative can be quite taxing. Speaking about a particular cover-up, Frank (England) explained:

> The thing is once I'd told that lie, I didn't realize how far the lie would go 'cos then you're constantly lying and the thing is I can never remember telling people things, I know I told them something but I can never remember what. ...[Plus,] you're constantly having to up-grade your lies.

Not only was constant lying burdensome; for many, it was something that contradicted the cultural model for close relationships. Many said that all close contacts should know they were HIV positive and accept them as such. HIV, said Jamie (England) is "something what makes me *me*." People who disclosed to assert identity were not necessarily seeking support from friends – just the acknowledgement that they were still themselves and the assurance that close contacts would see through the stigma. They were prepared to risk the dangers of self-disclosure to affirm their own identities, at least to their closest contacts.

In Western society, self-actualization and personal identity assertion have become important goals. Friendships and, especially, conjugal partnerships are ideal arenas in which to achieve them due to the expectation for self-development that such relationships entail (Cancian 1987). By definition and ideally, today, at least in our culture, close contacts are people with whom one can be oneself and the closer one is with a given individual the more personal information one should be able to share without threat of being rejected. Emotional and factual self-disclosures also are key factors in the development of intimacy and attachment (Laurenceau *et al.* 1998; Reis and Shaver 1988).

In general, the more distant the contact the less crucial asserting identity is in relation to the contact's need to know, as PHAs perceived it. There were, however, a number of exceptions to this rule, in which social distance did not play a part in decisions for or against self-disclosure of an AIDS identity. One Scotsman, for example, preferred not to work rather than 'live a lie' at work by not disclosing – even though those he worked with were not considered by him to be close contacts. Another raised money for charity by organizing a very public gambling pool on whether or not he would survive another year with HIV.

A few participants chose to disclose as part of public education campaigns, and often this dovetailed with a desire to avoid having to pretend to be seronegative. For example, five in the Scottish sample of 66 had appeared on television, in newspapers, or at AIDS conferences and disclosed to the public in efforts to decrease discrimination and increase awareness and resources for people with HIV. Others disclosed to challenge what they saw as ignorance. Betty, an IDU, said:

> See if I am sitting and people slag people with the virus and I will end up saying something. I will say like, "You don't know what you are fucking talking about. *I've got it!*" They have been pally [friendly] with me and they have touched me and they have drunk out of my cup and that, and I love doing that to people. They think they can tell by looking at somebody that they have got it. Like you go all thin and that. They go, "You are just kidding" or "You have not got it." I like doing it to people like that.

Immediate need

Most PHAs told someone about their condition upon diagnosis. About three-quarters of the Scottish participants told at least one person about their HIV status immediately after being diagnosed. This was almost always someone trusted and close, usually a partner or family member or a good friend. Others waited a week or two, but it was unusual to wait much longer. Still, four people in the Scottish sample (6%) told nobody for over a year.[11]

The motivation for telling at least one person directly after diagnosis was generally explained by reference to an almost irresistible need to tell — an urge to talk things through and to obtain support. For many, self-disclosure was relatively spontaneous albeit selective as, for example, for those who told a companion being tested at the same time, or for most of the people with haemophilia. The latter routinely gave parents or partners a report of their hospital visit anyhow, and those being tested together would be relatively prepared to hear such news.

Other disclosures were more considered, such as that of Gary, an 'out' gay Scotsman who disclosed to his six closest friends in the two or three days following his diagnosis. He trusted them, was confident that they would react well, and knew he needed their support to come to terms with his diagnosis. Similarly, Jamie (England) said to himself:

> "Who can I go and see?" So I went to see [a friend who worked for an AIDS service organization], a chap called [Joe], and his reaction, looking back, was exactly right. He didn't, "Oh you poor thing" or make a great

> sort of emotional turmoil out of it. He said "I will ring [Jack]" ... [a mutual friend] who is HIV positive ... and I spoke to him on the phone and he said "Oh you will be alright, don't worry about it. Wait till I get back home we will have a talk, bye." I thought "Oh well here we are."

Many participants recalled similarly calm responses from disclosees. In many cases, calmness or good reception seemed to us to be a result of successfully 'testing the water' (Limandri 1989) before disclosing.

Notwithstanding, many participants also recalled initial reactions of shock, and generally this came from contacts that the participant told because they felt they had to and not because of a feeling that those persons might be good persons to tell. For example, Robbie, an incarcerated Scottish IDU, recalled that his mother and sister were "just shattered, shattered," an expression used repeatedly by many of the Scottish sample.

Shock was not necessarily perceived as a bad reaction (most respondents had been shocked by their diagnoses themselves). Indeed, shock can be taken by a PHA to signify that others do not see him or her as "the type who would get AIDS," thus affirming his or her moral personhood.

Often, shock was followed by a positive affirmation of support. One-quarter of respondents in the Scottish study reported that a close contact to whom they had disclosed had arranged to visit a clinician treating the respondent or contacted an AIDS support agency to become better informed about the illness.[12] It was often reported, in such cases, that close contacts adapted well, came to terms with the illness and offered appropriate support.

In the majority of cases, respondents reported that the people to whom they had disclosed reacted well and supportively. Some of the reactions deemed most helpful involved touch rather than words; touch conveyed a sense of sympathy and no fear of contagion. For example, Gina, a Scot, told her sister who was a nurse as "she knows a bit about it and she just put her arms 'round me."

Organized support seeking

One response to diagnosis, and the sense of isolation that often accompanies it, is to make contact with HIV organisations and other people who have been diagnosed. Jamie (England) and Gary (Scotland), the gay-identified men discussed above, already knew some people in this capacity. But even those not involved in the gay community and those unfamiliar with HIV may reach out. Once one is a member of a support group or otherwise linked into a PHA community, friend-ships may flourish due to the shared experience of having the same disease and sometimes they become extremely close and enriching by virtue of this. As Vicky (Scotland) said, "Just knowing that you are not alone and that there is other people and you make friends. ...You become a lot stronger. I was not always this strong."

Whilst this type of bonding is generally reported as a very positive experience, the physical deterioration and death of new-found friends with HIV is extremely harrowing. George (Scotland) told us, "In the last two years I have been to about 12 funerals." Chuck (England) said:

I see people that ... they look really ill and all that and I look at myself in the mirror and I think you could be like that in six months' time you know, you just go – I think maybes it's that, it's just the fact of all these, oh, in [North-East location] you hear of a bloody funeral every other week you know what I mean.

While stories about meeting other PHAs sometimes involve negative feelings about future physical deterioration and death, they also can contain self-protective claims of superiority in terms of social status and moral characteristics. Said Malcolm of people he had met via service organisations in North-East England:

I only speak to them really because, I mean if I didn't know about them and they didn't know about me and I never went to this group, I don't know, we've got nothing in common. ...Some of them I don't trust, some of them have got prison records and other of them – I mean like some real weird people. ...One of them got accused of being a paedophile and I'm thinking they're not the sort of people I want to hang around with and they're not the sort of people I want to bring to my house. ...Some of 'em are real dodgy [questionable] characters.

So while support could be had through friendship with other PHAs, many found that simply sharing a disease was not enough to offset dissimilarities and social distance. Most of the participants did not care for group meetings. As Meg (USA) explained, "I shy away from support groups ... I don't want to tell strangers that I have HIV."

That's what friends and family are for

While contact with PHAs could offset isolation, most participants counted more on family and friends for support. Participants said that support during a major life event was one of the main things that family and friends were for, and disclosing to them to enlist their support often came 'naturally'.

Just as we did not limit the category of conjugal partner by requiring marriage or heterosexuality, we did not limit inclusion in the category of 'family' to those who were blood kin. Participants' own constructions of 'family' or 'friends' were respected and, although members did not always fit traditional criteria, the models participants held for family and friends, like the model held for conjugal relations (see below and Chapter 9), were fairly mainstream. For example, many felt it was their duty to inform close friends of major life events, as such sharing of information was a necessary part of having close friendships. According to Cathy (Scotland) "It is not a close friendship if you can't tell somebody because it is holding so much back from the friendship."

Frank (England) described telling a very close friend after a delay not warranted by his model (and his friend's) of friendship. The friend "was a bit upset because he wasn't told straight away he was sort of like the third or fourth person down the line to be told and ... he says, 'Who else knows?' and I told him and he said, 'Well why didn't you tell me?'" The two held a model of friendship that would have promoted earlier disclosure and by not disclosing early Frank jeopardized the relationship. But Frank may have felt damned if he did and damned if he didn't, knowing that the friend might have rejected him completely on the basis of his seropositivity. Because of the meaning of AIDS, the fragile boundary between safety and danger cannot be ensured even by friendship.

People reasoned that if close friends who were told did not react supportively then they were clearly, according to Morag, "not pals in the first place." Telling friends helped sort 'quality' friends from those who were not, and a high quality of relationship was seen as desirable, practically indispensable, to coping with HIV and to forming a positive identity as a person with HIV.

Participants reported that some relationships that had been stagnant or otherwise not ideal improved following disclosure, and that they now enjoyed much closer relationships than previously with some people. As Mick (Scotland) said, "Me and my father used to do fisticuffs, beat the hell out of each other. Now he hugs me, he loves me. I know he has always loved me but now he loves me more and he is showing it." Most participants said they took increased pleasure from the company of their closest contacts, valued quality not quantity of friendships, and in the words of Thomas, "put more effort into the ones that matter."

Sometimes, albeit rarely, a PHA disclosed while in the supportive friend or relation role rather than as a seeker of support. For friendship and kinship entails giving as well as accepting support from others, and people in healthy relationships normally swap these roles regularly. Said Chuck (England):

> I told [close family member] because she's [got an eating disorder] she had – and I really tried to get her to talk to her and I told her that she was killing herself and I said, "Listen [Jane] I'm not very well," and she says, "There's nothing wrong with you." I says, "Well there is actually," I says, "You're killing yourself and I'm feel as though I'm dying," I said, "with no control of my own," so I you know – and that actually did have a great impact on her 'cos she changed her way-like a bit. She hasn't got it now. It took her about a year but I think it done some sort of good like that.

Love, trust, and partnership

Just as friendship ideals and ideals for family relations provide some of the bases for disclosure guidelines, participants appealed to longstanding mainstream conjugal constructs when discussing their feelings regarding disclosure to primary sexual partners. Mainstream relationship ideals highlight trust and honesty (Sobo 1993a, 1995b), and in light of this, nondisclosure implies duplicity or at least a failure to honour the foundations of trust that conjugal relations are built upon. In a statement that conveyed his feelings about relationship ideals as well as making a claim about where he stood on a moral scale in relation to others who did not honour those ideals, Frank (England) said:

> There's this er magazine that I have I've sometimes picked up. It's called *Positive Nation*, and I've picked up articles in there and people have been positive and their partners haven't known and they haven't told them for like 5 or 10 years and I've sat there thinking ... if you love somebody and you're in a relationship you share everything with them and you know you've got to trust – if there's no trust there's no point in having a relationship in my eyes.

Similarly, Kevin, the only English participant in a relationship with a woman at the time of interview said, "I have hid silly little things [but seropositivity] is too big an issue I think to hide from your partner ... I love her and I wouldn't want to hurt her by deceiving her, I think I would be deceiving her." He added, "She would probably wonder why I wanted to wear a condom all the time." Kevin claimed with this addition that he would protect his partner in any case from the risk of HIV transmission, positioning himself again as someone who respected the conjugal ideal for altruistic self-sacrifice for the partner's benefit.

As Jamie (England) explained, "I think you reach a point in a relationship where you have built up sufficient trust in each other ... I think you would end up being underhand and deceitful." Jamie's claim about deceit involves an implicit theory about how relationships evolve. A relationship reaches a stage where trust has been "built up," and it is at this stage that nondisclosure becomes a problem. Further, if this stage is nearing, disclosure can serve as a catalyst, pushing the relationship into the latter category, cementing previously casual bonds.

Jamie said of the beginning of a previous long-term partnering:

> I knew that my feelings for [previous partner] were quite strong and I wanted to keep on seeing him, I wanted him to be part of my life. ...[The HIV is] an important thing about me, and so to hide that or to leave that to one side would just imply dishonesty or would imply "I don't trust you" or "I don't think you are worthy of knowing this about me" ... [His] reaction was "I knew you were going to say that, don't worry about it." ... It was a lovely reaction, there was no negativity there. [I told him] probably after and before [sex ...] 'cos it is a sort of intimate time and yeah.

Jamie used the intimacy of sex to set the stage for his intimate, identity-related disclosure. Sharing such personal details – meeting relationship ideals by being so honest and trusting and providing his partner with an opportunity to demonstrate that he too could meet relationship ideals for supportiveness and unconditional loving – brought the couple to a more certain union.

While all of the above examples of love, trust and partnership are from North-East England, participants at each site expressed similar ideals. We return to intimate disclosure in Chapter 9. But before we go into detail about specific types of self-disclosure, we need to discuss the dangers that disclosure can entail. In the present chapter, we've discussed disclosure broadly, observing some of its general benefits and the contexts in which it seems to work well. We discussed the cultural ideals that people use when assessing whether self-disclosure to certain categories of people is warranted. Cultural models come into play in the next chapter too, which examines the main reasons people give when they do not want to self-disclose, and the risk-assessment process they use in coming to the decision to remain silent about what for many is seen as a dangerous side of the self.

Notes

1 They may of course have looked unwell to people who knew them well.

2 Comparison statistics are not available from the English or American data.

3 Limandri (1989) also found that sometimes, especially when knowing about one's condition causes great stress, self-disclosure can be "venting" (i.e. compulsive or explosive).

4 Many PHAs in our samples talked about the process of risk assessment as a cost-benefit exercise. Most PHAs in our studies (but by no means all) received counselling about disclosure at time of testing or shortly afterwards. Perhaps as a result of exposure to the counselling vocabulary, or maybe because the participants are heirs to the same "industrial habits of mind" (Adam 1998: 58) as those that lead scholars to the limited conceptualization of risk that we critiqued in Chapter 3, many PHAs in our samples talked about the process of risk assessment as a cost-benefit exercise.

5 While cultural ideals may posit that kin should be closer than friends should and one's married partner should be closest of all, people's personal continuums varied just as their lifestyles did. For example, many gays in particular, did not seem to feel as close to their families as they did to their friends. Further, many felt as close to their primary paraconjugal partners as they would have if they were married to them. Many had causal sexual partners to whom they felt no closeness. Social intimacy is the key to the continuum but sexual intimacy does not necessarily translate into that. We deal with disclosure to sexual partners in more depth in Chapters 9 and 10.

6 We drew on Sobo (1997), with kind permission, in writing this section on moral discourse.

7 The narrative construction of oneself as a culturally respectable and moral being is a collaborative inter-subjective process. Further, it is a process in which people think about what others are thinking about them. That is, when we converse we are not simply telling stories but reacting to reactions, both real and imagined, on the part of our conversational partners or interlocutors. We anticipate our conversational partner's thoughts, interpret his or her actual reactions, and respond in ways that we perceive of as appropriate. In other words, and as MacIntyre notes, "We are never more (and sometimes less) than the co-authors of our own narratives" (1985: 213). Co-authoring occurs between particular individuals in relation to the particular intentions and read intentions of those individuals or interlocutors and, ultimately, to culturally shared paradigmatic models of moral action. Together, interlocutors create each other as good (or bad) people, using culturally constructed models as "coherence mechanisms" for condensing and reifying as a self or an identity certain actions, intentions or experiences (de Munck 1992: 182).

8 General, overarching moral models can come into play during story-telling and conversation, but more often people deploy the lower level models embedded in these (regarding cultural models and their motivating force, see D'Andrade 1992; Quinn and Holland 1987; Strauss 1992).

9 In the following chapter (Chapter 7) we examine situations, e.g. the casual sexual encounter, in which this moral imperative to disclose is overridden by other concerns.

10 Some did, however, argue that they could perhaps cut themselves and thus place others at risk.

11 Similar quantitative data are not available for the other sites.

12 Similar quantitative data are not available for the other sites.

The danger of disclosure

When others know too much

Despite the many reasons for disclosing – providing protection, identity assertion, laying claim to support, confirming friendship, family, and love relations – disclosing has many potential dangers. Similar statements regarding dangers were recorded at all three sites and any differences had more to do with mode of transmission or individual biography than with inter-site distinctions.

Double stigma

Many participants, particularly heterosexuals and haemophiliacs, were deterred from disclosing by the 'double stigma': the association of HIV with so-called high-risk groups and culturally disdained actions. Jack, a young Scot with haemophilia, told of an agreement he had made with his sister and parents "to keep the HIV between the four people in the house. ...They were worried about what other people would think. Things like I was a drug addict." Besides fearing double stigmatization, Jack saw that his stigma might be extended to them in what Goffman called a 'courtesy' (1963).

For some, the threat of double stigma was so great that they questioned the origin of their infection. Derek (Scotland) said he had taken part in no risk behaviour whatsoever and did not know how he had become infected, claiming that there had to be an unknown mode of transmission. Whilst this is a theoretical possibility, it seems more likely that Derek could not bring himself to tell his seronegative wife or perhaps even himself that he had injected drugs or had extramarital sex.

Derek's position was not unique. Even people that self-identified as members of stigmatized groups and those who freely described participation in risky activity would often state that their infections were flukes. Disavowals of promiscuity were commonly seen in the data from North-East England. Members of the sample said, for example, "I don't know if I contracted it via sexual contact, it would have been fairly difficult 'cos I've always followed safer sex practice;" "The one time I caught the virus it was just a one-off job. ... I never done nothing you know what I mean? ... I suppose I was one of the unlucky ones wasn't I?"; "I'd always practised safer sex, so I just figured well just my bloody luck i'nt it? Kiss of death."

Frank described his lack of risky behaviour and the subsequent grilling he got from the doctor who diagnosed him:

> Quite honestly I didn't feel that I had done anything what had put me at risk ... like either having anal intercourse or, or injecting drugs, I've never done any of that so I couldn't suss out where I, you know where I'd actually picked the virus up from. ...He [the doctor] said to me, I can't remember what term he used but he said something like em, "Do you shoot up?" And I went, "I beg your pardon?" He went, "Can I have a look at you arms?" And I went, "Yes, what do you mean?" And he had a look at my arms; he says, "You're not a drug user are you?" I went, "No." ..."So you've never em injected yourself?" I went, "No." ...So em he says, "Right, have you ever been with a prostitute?" "No." He says, "Have you ever had unprotected penetrative sex?" I went, "No," and he sat there and he says, "Well I'm confused," he said "You're obviously lying to me." I went, "Why?" I said, "What have I got to gain by lying to you, you're my doctor. You're not my mother you're my doctor."

That confessing to such actions would have implicated him as immoral is made clear by Frank's reference to the mother role when chastizing the doctor for his incredulity.

Testimony from the English sample was cut through with denials of immorality and statements dissociating oneself from 'regular' PHAs (more of which later). The stigma of AIDS was enough itself without having to cope with the stigma of being promiscuous or incautious.[1]

Double disclosure

Those deterred by the fear of double stigmatization included those who defined themselves as members of one or another 'risk group' and preferred to keep such membership hidden, at least from some of their social contacts. Jim, a gay Scot, was unable to disclose his HIV status to his father as he felt this would necessitate also disclosing his gay identity, an identity he feared his father would be unable to accept. Gary, another gay Scot, felt unable to tell his dentist of many years standing he was HIV positive as this would require revealing too much of his personal identity; he preferred to seek a dentist elsewhere.

In a statement that expressed fear of double stigma and courtesy stigma too, as well as a desire to protect his mother, in fitting with kinship ideals, Chuck (England) explained:

> The reason why I moved away and come to university and everything is because where [I lived] it's so small and, and people are so narrow minded that if they found out that if that her son had died of this she'd have to move. ...So, it's not fair on my mum to be put through that so I figured if nobody knows and I could like say it was actually "Oh your son died of cancer" or something like that, well then she would still be acceptable in the village. Now if they found out her son died of, it would be like, they'd be painting bloody red crosses on her door ... and putting a bell round her neck. If anybody found out I was gay let alone eventually "Oh he died of AIDS" my mother would have to like leave, leave the village and move off, they'd either stone her or like paint a, walk 'round with a cow bell 'round my neck saying 'unclean' or something like that. ...So em, I was doing it [keeping it secret] like on a protection kind of thing.

Disbelief

Especially for people who do not fit AIDS stereotypes – for those who are not IDUs or gay men – another barrier exists: disbelief. Even those who should know better – AIDS service providers and other PHAs – can express disbelief. Bob (England), a heterosexual, was accused of pulling "a big hoax-like" when he walked into a regional service centre looking for help; "They thought, 'No he is just cunning-like. He doesn't belong here'" because he did not fit the proper image of the PHA.[2]

Gina, from Glasgow, lamented that her boyfriend refused to accept her diagnosis. "He thought I was telling him that because I didn't want to see him anymore, that I wanted to end the relationship and he couldn't believe, no way that I could have picked up HIV, I wasn't that kind of girl basically." Some participants explained sexual partners' refusal to believe as based in what they called "[AIDS-risk] denial", a term that they used as if self-explanatory.[3] The following interchange is from a New Mexico focus group:

Rick: I've had people say to me, "Well, you don't have AIDS; you don't need to use a condom." I said "Regardless of what I am, you would use a condom wouldn't you?" ...Not only are they loose, but ...

Dee: They think we too healthy to have AIDS. If you're overweight you don't have anything.

Ron: You've got to be skinny, have your hair falling out or something.

Dee: I tell them, "You don't realize! You need to get more educated on that subject ... " I have said to people, "Why do you want to be with me? For all you know I got AIDS!" [And they say,] "Oh look at you: all them big thighs! You don't have any AIDS." They're in denial.

Participants talk about the problem of disbelief and at the same time they position themselves as responsible people, in contrast to the 'loose' and rather careless people they have encountered sexually.

More common than a response of total denial was the disclosee's simple refusal to deal with the information. Vicky (Scotland) was a heavily pregnant teenager and with her mother when she received her diagnosis. She said that her mother was not able to deal with the diagnosis at the time or subsequently:

Vicky: She made me get the bus home and that and was saying like "Pull yourself together" and that, like "Everybody is looking at you" ... I remember going home and she made me sit at the tea table and eat my tea and things like that. "You have got to eat to keep your strength up like because you are pregnant." ...

GG: So do you just not talk to her about HIV?

Vicky: I have tried a few times, but I know for sure that there is no way I am going to get through.

Many PHAs reported telling friends or family and then never again speaking frankly with them about their diagnosis. Some felt that, in the words of one Scot, "they shun away from the subject." This was reported with regret although the participants generally acknowledged that they felt reticent too. As Mitch (Scotland) said, "I do not talk to [my mother] about it. It is not something that you really talk about."

Being unable to talk to close contacts about HIV can be a source of, or something that adds to, frustration and isolation. Distancing from closest contacts may occur even if they have been disclosed to and are supportive in other respects.

Coddling treatment

While silence could be disheartening, many participants were afraid of over-attentive responses. They dreaded being treated with "kid gloves," or offered "tea and sympathy." Malcolm (England) explained why: "Attitudes can be really disempowering and em independence robbing ... I'm not in the grave yet ... please don't treat me as though I'm wrapped in cotton wool because I will bop you [laughs]."

Kevin (England) told a story demonstrating how much extra emotional work people's coddling can involve for PHAs:

> I watched *Eastenders* [a UK TV soap] the other night where Peggy laid into Mark about his being HIV and things and [my friends] are all sitting there looking at me. I am sitting there fine with my cup of coffee and my cigarette, [girlfriend] has got tears running out of her eyes, [friend's] got tears running out of his eyes and [second friend is] nearly crying. I said "What's the matter with yous?" They said "Aaah." I said "I'm fine man, I'm cush." "You are going to die." "I am not going to die, I still have got loads of years left in me to give you grief." Then that just made them laugh.

The burden placed on others

Beside concern over being treated "like an invalid", participants worried about upsetting others. Disclosure was often withheld from parents and other close family members, at least until one's health deteriorated, in order to save them from worry. People with HIV may thus exclude themselves from the family's potential as a source of support, as the following interchange with Marie, a young Scottish IDU who came from a large Catholic family, shows.

Marie: I had sort of made lists in my mind who I could tell, who I would tell and who I could tell but would get too upset so I am not going to tell them. That kind of list.

GG: And how did you decide which ones?

Marie: Just how I knew they would react.

GG: And which was the longest list?

Marie: Who I could tell but would be too upset, that is most of my family including my ma and da.

Losing information control

A fear of gossip also figures prominently in disclosure decision-making. All participants were aware that the more people they told of their HIV status the less control they had over the management of this information. A casual partner's potential role as a gossip was horrifying to Janie (USA), whose whole family learned of her illness through the grapevine. Still, as she knew, people often cannot help talking; when Janie told one confidant, "it affected her and she had to tell [someone else] so she could help herself".

Even people expected to respond supportively were sometimes not told because participants feared they might tell others. This included some of the participants' children, who were not told lest they passed the information on to others. And some even felt the threat of exposure from other PHAs. Jamie (England) said, "I've tended to be nice to [PHAs from the support group] even though I don't particularly want to be nice to them 'cos I was that scared of what they could turn round and say to other people."

There were a number of instances in which participants felt they had very little control from the outset about the management of information about their HIV status. Bill, a Scottish IDU, was informed of his diagnosis in a room with an open door and the 20 prisoners in the adjoining room overheard. Chuck (England) learned of his diagnosis in hospital; the doctor "come bouncing in through the open ward and he come bouncing 'round my bed and whipped the curtains 'round and went 'Oh sorry but you're HIV positive'" for all the ward to hear. There were also cases of professionals telling participants' parents about their diagnoses. In addition, small seemingly inconsequential incidents such as receiving a letter from an infectious disease clinic or a visit from a health worker were often sufficient to generate gossip among those who sorted incoming mail or noticed visitors' arrivals.

Participants were aware that once several people knew of their serostatus there was always a chance it could become more widely known. About one-third of those interviewed in Glasgow, for whom we have such quantitative data, felt that information about their serostatus had largely been placed out of their control.

Many disclosees who had been asked by participants to keep silent broke confidence and told others. According to the participants, some disclosees needed the support of others to deal with the information, others felt that other people had a right to know, and others could not resist sharing such rich material for gossip. Some 'let it slip' unintentionally or in answer to a direct question, and some told others out of malice.

The way in which information about an individual's HIV status can spread amongst a circle of friends was seen in Vanessa's (Scotland) reflection on who in her circle knew her status. She said, "I think [Clara] has got a rough idea that I am positive somehow. But she has not come out and said it you know. [Karl] knows because [Jan] or [Harry] told him. ...[And Steven] thinks he may have told [Norma] and if so she might have told [Marie]."

The fear that disclosure may lead to one's information spreading out of control appears well founded. Participants often felt hurt that a trusted affiliate had disappointed them. Nonetheless, information spread was occasionally perceived as an advantage as it saved participants from the agony and embarrassment disclosure can entail. And it could be an advantage for other reasons too; for example, Vanessa's boyfriend told his mother, "and she just went like that 'I always knew that lassie wasn't well'. ...She told him to treat me better. She will say to him 'and I hope you are not lifting your hands [in violence] to that lassie'."

Things did not go so smoothly for John (Scotland), who told his brother one night and asked him not to tell his wife:

> So we had a meal and later on the two of them [his brother and sister-in-law] were in the kitchen doing the dishes and I heard her scream. He had told her. ... I felt bad about that. I saw no reason for him to tell her. ... Anyway like the kids were going to bed and my young nephew came over and kissed me goodnight and I could see her standing and quite literally pulling hair out of her head.

To the sister-in-law, John's dangerousness and his potential to harm her children was manifest, although in time she came to terms with John's diagnosis and welcomed him into her home.

As Lorrie, a gay Scot, reported, when information spreads beyond PHAs' immediate social circles, they may have to deal with "wee [little] secret call outs, 'I heard he's got AIDS'." The feeling that people are talking behind one's back was common. Peter (Scotland), a heterosexual with haemophilia, said that an acquaintance of his "would tell people I didn't really know, especially females so that they would not go near me". Mick (Scotland) reported a similar response from a female friend: "She's been saying to people I've got AIDS, 'don't be his lover', 'don't do this', 'don't touch him', you know. It hurts."

Gossip was just as problematic in the gay community or on the 'gay scene' as elsewhere. Malcolm (England) said:

> I had an expectation with HIV being much more prevalent here and sort of much bigger in the gay population that there'd be support from the gay community and in the meantime the gay community's almost rabidly anti-HIV; well if someone is HIV positive the last thing they should do is disclose on the scene ... they will tear you, shoot you down in flames.

Chuck, who was very involved in the North-East England 'scene', was once invited by a service provider to participate in an event that would implicate him as a PHA.

> They said "We're having a, a day seminar where people from the local gay pubs and that the managers and manageresses they're going to be there as well." And I said, "There's no way I'm turning up there," I said, "I know these people, they can't keep anything quiet," I said, "If I turned up there and they saw me within an hour my name would be mud!"

According to Jamie, at least in North-East England, "The scene is very orientated towards youth and looks" and the 'body beautiful'. In this, the scene is similar to that which Stall (1997) has described for the San Francisco area in the USA, where the pressure to look young and fit is very high, compounding the social risk of illness or disability. The centre of a gay scene can be a very risky place to be ugly or ill in. Matthew, one of the youngest English interviewees, said:

> I only heard about this but a few people that were getting ill and getting signs of being ill and all that, withdrawn face around the cheekbones and all sorts and like dry skin ... went in [a particular gay pub] once or twice and people wouldn't speak to them, they wouldn't go anywhere near

them so they haven't been back. [That pub] in a way is like an AIDS-free zone.

Matthew's preface, "I only heard about this," is important: he had not experienced this type of response himself. Nonetheless, he had learned through stories to anticipate it.

Rejection

Many participants feared that a serostatus disclosure would fundamentally alter relationships and change people's views of them. This went even for AIDS service volunteers and professionals (see Chapter 8). Janie (USA) said, "When the volunteers help you, they look at you, and you go, 'Oh, God, now if you ever see me on the street you're going to know'"; "You have to go get your prescription and then the pharmacist knows what this prescription is for, and ... you go, 'Oh God, they know'."

The fear that a relationship would change upon disclosure was particularly acute when making decisions about disclosure to those that mattered most, such as one's children or a new partner. Many participants spoke of the anguish they experienced telling a new potential long-term sexual partner; one woman in the Scottish sample reported it had driven her to attempt suicide. Another Scottish woman, Heather, was unable to tell her partner even when he insisted that they stop using condoms. She said, "I don't know why but I was scared to open up to him. Once he found some HIV leaflets and he went, 'Have you got AIDS?' I said, 'No,' and I just could not say anything. ...I felt really guilty about this."

The risk of rejection was the most commonly given reason for non-disclosure; at the same time, stories of full, all-out rejection from people who mattered to the PHAs were rare. But they were not entirely absent. Lorrie (Scotland) described immediate rejection from a lover:

> As soon as he walked in the door I sat him down with a cup of tea and poured him a large brandy. I said "You'll need that as well" and I told him and two hours later he had his suitcases packed and walked out. ...He just disappeared straight out of the door.

Most rejections were far less dramatic and took the form of a gradual winding down of a friendship which, as most participants acknowledged, may have happened anyhow.

Partial rejections were more common. Many participants reported incidents in which others made them feel dangerous. Thomas (Scotland) recounted being reprimanded by his sister while sharing a bowl of strawberries:

> You know how you take a strawberry and you put it in the sugar and then you eat it and then you do it again. She said, "What about your saliva?" and stuff like that quite hurt me. I said, "You can't catch it off saliva." She said, "Don't do that anyway it's a dirty habit." She has never pulled me up for stuff like that before.

What is most striking about the data from each site is that total rejection of the PHA, particularly from close contacts, was extremely rare. This may reflect the accurate judgement of the PHA about who to disclose to, although rejection was also unusual among friends and family members who had found out about a PHA's HIV status indirectly, e.g. from a third party. The rare cases of outright rejection mainly came from distant acquaintances rather than close friends. This may reflect the redrawing of friendship lines by PHAs following disclosure. According to commonly held cultural understandings about friendship, no true friend would react so negatively, a friend who rejects a PHA may in retrospect be classified as always having been a distant acquaintance, and never having been a real friend after all.

Rejection or discrimination was, however, occasionally reported from strangers. Bob, a Scotsman with haemophilia, reported discrimination during two job interviews in which he mentioned he was HIV-positive.

Bob: We had a little talk about medical matters and then I was in-between whether to tell them I had HIV or not tell them and I thought well I'll try it and see what happens and on both occasions it got a very cold reception, very cold.

GG: In what way did they become cold?

Bob: Their attitude changed. It was a kind of rolling interview and going along quite well and then all of a sudden it became broken, staccatoed kind of thing, humming and hahing and saying "oh well eh" – that kind of thing but I mean they were very nice but they always are, you know, when they are about to say no anyway.

In the second job interview, initially he disclosed only his haemophilia.

> And we talked about it for a few minutes and it was fine, you know. He then says, "Wasn't there something to do with haemophiliacs being HIV?" So I took it that he was interested in the subject and he would be quite

sympathetic towards it you know and [I] asked whether HIV is a question they ask when hiring in the company or something like that. Of course as soon as I opened my mouth I knew I'd done the wrong thing. He looked at me as though I'd hit him with a brick. ...He had made the link and that was it, it was gone. From that point it had gone.

While nothing was said verbally, Bob noted changes in attitude and ascribed the cause to his seropositivity. Similarly, Jane, an army wife, reported that her husband's career was ruined following her diagnosis, although he tested HIV-negative. He was confined to working in a restricted number of countries and his opportunities for advancement were severely restricted. Even if the restrictions had naught to do with courtesy stigmatization, the important point here is that Jane felt sure that they did.

Although overt rejection, real or perceived, was only rarely reported, fear of rejection permeated each sample. This fear was sometimes based upon painful previous experience but more often it was based on tales like the one Matthew had been told about the "AIDS-free" gay pub he described above.

Jamie (England), who realized early in his first interview that he had no real rejection stories of his own, still said, "Other people em, they've disclosed and they've had like lots of bad you know a lot of bad things have come from it, like their families haven't wanted anything to do with them and they've been a real close knit family before."

Calculating risks

Are reactions as bad as PHAs expect?

Discrimination does happen and three participants across all three research sites said that they had personally experienced what they would define as hate crime. In general, though, and no doubt partly due to the screening process that usually precedes deciding to disclose, rejection from close contacts was rare. Still, while some people felt quite relaxed about disclosure as a result of good reaction experiences, the majority of respondents felt very uncomfortable indeed about disclosure and they generally preferred to keep their HIV identity hidden. For example, Scottish haemophiliac Jack said, "It's like with racism and homophobia you just don't know with people." Jack told no one outside his family circle. His life became very restricted as a result: he kept few social contacts, had no sexual partners and had no work.

Fear of rejection notwithstanding, most PHAs we spoke with tended to have better reactions from disclosees than they expected. It therefore seems likely that there is a general tendency for PHAs to overestimate the stigma of being HIV positive (a finding supported by data discussed in later chapters as well). Why do PHAs have a tendency to overestimate the social risk of being HIV positive?

Fear of bad reactions and stigma are, in part, fuelled by shared understandings that the behaviours associated with AIDS are not culturally condoned. Even those who condone street drug use or gay anal sex seem not to condone what they define as promiscuity (a relative term) and they disavow, in their own infection stories, bad behaviour on their own part – behaviour that they know 'the public' often links with PHAs.

Moreover, media images of PHAs that were prominent just prior to the years of this research tended to focus upon the most horrific aspects of the virus and of people with it. Jamie (England) said:

> When you read kind of like scare stories and tabloid articles you sort of think this is about me in some way. ...I think perhaps in some sort of subtle way I perhaps internalize some of the negativities that come across in articles like that and think, you know, I am walking around with this horrible virus inside me.

And the virus does not always hide inside. Malcolm (England) explained that "Although HIV was internal and invisible, I felt that it was very visible as well; sort of I felt that people could see."

In addition to tabloid stories, PHAs are faced with health promotion messages that focus upon the late stages of the disease or images of death such as tombstones. As Timothy (England) observed, "We're not really encouraged to see that HIV people can be productive healthy members of society we sort of, we see ... Kaposis ravaged faces glaring out of posters." Jamie (England) said that knowledge of the public image of AIDS "is quite a burden to carry around and certainly it makes it an uphill battle having a positive self image."

Newspapers reported arson attacks on the homes of people with AIDS, educational exclusion for children with AIDS due to the reaction of the parents of their classmates, and many other types of discrimination against people with AIDS. As Malcolm (England) noted, "you sort of take on board other people's paranoias." In this climate, local stories about reactions to people with HIV became distorted. This was clearly demonstrated in the Scottish study.

Two young brothers with haemophilia were infected with HIV. Their father campaigned for compensation and as part of this struggle the boys came to the attention of the local and national media. Many study participants with haemophilia (who were annoyed that this publicity had clearly spelled out the link between HIV and haemophilia) reported that the family had as a result been subjected to persecution from their neighbours. As Donald, who lived in a rural area not far from the brothers, said:

> There is two lads that live near us, well used to live near us. I think they have moved away now because they were spat on at school and they were haemophiliacs and they had unfortunately picked this [HIV] up. They were treated like bloody lepers awful you know. The family had to move out of the area because of local press and things. It was horrific.

But what had really happened? One of the brothers in the story, Pat, was in the study sample. According to him, after his family 'went public' he received only supportive reactions from his neighbours and school. He said that the town's Council had wanted to move the family into a larger house but they said they would prefer to build an extension to their dwelling. The neighbours all signed a petition to support their staying there. Another family member organized a petition in the area asking for compensation for haemophiliacs. They collected 20,000 signatures from the small town where they were living and reported a very sympathetic response from the local people.

In stark contrast to most of the participants with haemophilia, Pat felt that most people are sympathetic towards PHAs and do not behave in a stigmatizing manner. He explained this attitude as the result of his own very positive experience.

Shifting landscapes of risk

Fear of being rejected was common to all participants and most recognised the enormous hurt and damage to self-esteem and identity that rejection would cause. Whilst a few had the self-confidence to reason, like Thomas (Scotland), that "if they don't like it and don't accept me as I am then I don't need them", at the time of interview few were as self-assured.

Still, the context in which disclosure risk assessments are made may change dramatically according to factors such as health, number of people who have already been told, previous experience of disclosing, etc. It was common, for example, for participants to disclose to a wider circle of people when they became symptomatic or were hospitalized. This was partly because as the illness advanced it became more physically apparent; previously only 'discreditable', PHAs now became 'discredited', in Goffman's (1963) terms.

PHAs with advancing symptoms reasoned that people would soon find out anyway, and being ill with HIV tended then to become a central identity factor. Also, when illness took over, participants feared that the hurt close friends or relatives might feel at being excluded (uninformed) would be a greater relationship danger than their concern and worry or disapproval. Lorrie, a gay Scot, told his family when he was hospitalized and asked by a clinic staff member to name his next-of-kin. He felt they would be offended if he did not name them, "so the family had to be told".

Most of our interviewees were not so sick, and in most cases potential dangers deterred people from disclosure. With the exception of those who needed to have a public HIV-identity, such as those who were involved in campaign work, participants in our studies tended not to risk disclosure to those who did not need to know, as the potential dangers were almost always high. For instance, disclosing to a casual sexual partner, for example, may minimize guilt in the event of HIV transmission, or even reduce the chances of transmission by encouraging safer sex. However, such disclosure can potentially be met with rejection and the discloser can lose control of the management of information about his or her HIV status. A casual sexual partner is not as well known or trusted as a close friend and does not owe one the same level or kind of allegiance.

The landscape of risk in which disclosure decisions are made is constantly changing in response to a myriad of elements. On the local level, say the PHA becomes ill, finds a new partner, gets a new job, goes to prison, stops using drugs – any of these changes will radically alter the risk landscape. So too will local-level changes among their close contacts. One woman in the Scottish sample, for example, told how her risk landscape changed after her partner was diagnosed with a chronic illness unrelated to HIV. This changed the structure of their relationship (they now shared the caring role) and her assessment of social risk. She was far less bothered by who knew about her HIV status than she had formerly been and far more concerned about when and how her partner would disclose his own condition to his friends.

There are also higher-level changes that affect the risk landscape: a new therapy that seems to delay disease progression, a new film that challenges intolerance towards PHAs, a media story highlighting the dangerous identity of the PHA. Limitless local and global factors can contribute to each individual's landscape of risk. In Chapter 3, we described handling social risk in a shifting risk landscape as juggling a grand piano, an anvil and a feather on a storm-tossed boat in a turbulent sea; the factors which constitute the risk landscape are in continuous and unstoppable motion.

A process of risk assessment

The narratives offered by participants at all sites suggest that disclosure decision-making tends to be a carefully considered, rational process. In general, people with HIV consider both the pros and cons of disclosure before making their decisions. They take into account past experiences, and are influenced by their perception of the attitude of others towards PHAs. Those with no past experiences of their own to go by will still have heard second-hand or media accounts of what disclosure can lead to. Predicted future experiences may serve as an anchor in the PHA's calculus of risk.

For example, Michael, a young Scot, makes what appear to be situated rationality decisions based upon perceived need to know, closeness to the person, and an assessment of what their reaction to disclosure will be:

> Some people I definitely won't tell. People firstly that I think don't need to know. If there is people that don't need to know, I still tell some of them. I think the difference is how close to them or if it just happens to come out because we are having a heart to heart about something. They are just giving me a major heart to heart about their life sort of thing so I open up to them. Some people I don't tell because I think it would change too much their attitude of me. I don't want them to start worrying about me, I don't want to have that so I would not tell them.

Similar evidence of a 'calculus of risk' was plentiful in the decision-making narratives we collected. Notwithstanding, and as suggested in Chapter 3's discussion of the rhetoric of risk, participants may have exaggerated the rationality underlying disclosure decision-making. First, most PHAs in our samples had talked to counsellors, either at time of testing or shortly following, and in these sessions the issue of disclosure was generally discussed. In the knowledge that an HIV identity is socially dangerous, counsellors tend to encourage a cautious and rational approach to disclosure. PHAs are advised to consider carefully each individual in their network and identify whether or not they 'need to know' and what their reactions are likely to be.

Thus, a rational considered approach to disclosure decision-making is encouraged at the outset as an appropriate model for newly diagnosed PHAs. It is therefore likely that when being interviewed by someone who in age and social position is not unlike a counsellor, PHAs will refer back to this model in their post-rationalizations about their disclosure decisions.

Such rationalism also is encouraged by habits of mind that industrialism brought about in the West (Adam 1998: 58) and which we discussed in Chapter 3.

117

Additionally, one's actions or decisions, in retrospect, have a tendency to become more rational in the telling, as we label and compartmentalize our pasts in our efforts to make sense of our worlds (see also MacIntyre 1985).

Disclosure decision-making may sometimes appear similar to a simple cost-benefit calculation exercise. But it is not actually that. First, unlike when figuring which potatoes are the better buy, the equations for figuring out to whom disclosure will be beneficial can have huge error margins which may have a long-term impact. Second, the variables that one must figure in are themselves constantly shifting. Disclosure decisions are set within the ever-changing risk landscape. While a complicated process of risk assessment accompanies a decision there is always an element of uncertainty. And, just as a betting man occasionally has a flutter on an outsider, the PHA may occasionally decide to risk disclosure despite an overall expectation of a negative outcome. Such risky behaviour tends to be relatively spontaneous and often is taken under the influence of alcohol or spurred by a crisis. In general it occurs in newer relationships, particularly sexual ones; the PHA, following widely available cultural models for friendship or conjugal relations, reasons that she has to disclose all in order for the relationship to develop, and to preserve 'his or her' own integrity and identity.

Other factors also suggest that not all disclosures follow a rational process. For instance, one-third of the sample in the Scottish study was tested without asking to be so and most of them received no counselling at time of testing (although many have since). This was most common among the more socially disadvantaged individuals in the study. Often understanding little about HIV or its consequences, many of those in this situation were in a disoriented state following diagnosis and any disclosures they made in the subsequent weeks followed no coherent or planned strategy.

And some people just chose not to follow the 'need to know' model. A Scottish motorcycle enthusiast, for example, told all his non-work contacts regardless of their closeness or 'need to know'. His identity as a biker appeared key: being HIV could be readily incorporated into his identity as a high-risk, fast-driving, hell-raiser and would not demean his status among his biker peers so long as he pitched it this way. The fact that he told none of his work associates for fear of being fired illustrates well the shifting and situational nature of risk landscapes and how, just as different facets of one's identity emerge in different settings, disclosure may be appropriate in one context but not in another.

The changeable nature of the risk landscape unfolds in the following chapters, which examine disclosure in two specific social arenas: health care and conjugal relations. Although both arenas entail bodily intimacy, relationships with health care workers are instrumental or pragmatic while those with sexual partners are expressive or emotion based. The next three chapters examine the differences entailed and link self-disclosure in these specific settings to a general theory of self-disclosure and social risk.

Notes

1   The stigma of being careless was perhaps especially feared in the UK, where AIDS education campaigns were pitched with the slogan, "Don't die of ignorance." Frank himself pointed this out, and he also observed of many PHAs he had met, "They don't want to confront the possibility that their behaviour, their sort of, where everyone's sort of, where people are promiscuous and I've sort of encountered it talking to people from time to time they sort of say 'I wasn't that promiscuous really' ... sort of a double blindness ... sort of like 'I wasn't that bad'."

2   Another heterosexual in the English sample said of the same organization, "[It] is for like gay people. ...Like they were sitting at the dining table having your meal and all the queens are having a laugh and if you try and [join] in you are sort of gently pushed to the sides as if to say, 'Who asked for your opinion?'"

3   However, some of the participants' comments regarding condom symbolism, a few examples of which we provide in Chapter 9, indicate some understanding of denial's psycho-cultural motivations. These have to do with the insult to self-esteem that condom use connotes (see Sobo 1993a, 1995b).

Chapter 8

Reported reactions in health care settings

The last two chapters discussed disclosure in general; we reviewed the main factors that figure in people's assessments of the social risk that sharing serostatus information may entail. In general, the more socially distant a person was from the PHA, the less likely the PHA was to disclose; this minimized rejection experiences. But there are certain socially distant people that PHAs must, in theory, disclose to: those who service their health-care needs. The 'need to know' attributed to health care workers (HCWs) is generally high due to the risk of infection (albeit small) associated with some health care procedures.[1]

Relations with HCWs are primarily instrumental or pragmatic rather than expressive or social. As HCWs are neither kith nor kin they cannot be expected to offer the same kind of support that friends and family should do. Social distance notwithstanding, PHAs may expect HCWs to be well informed about HIV and unbiased in their treatment of them. We have seen that disclosures to close social contacts do not necessarily conform to the negative expectations that PHAs have learned to have. How do experiences in health care settings compare?

HCWs and people with stigmatized conditions

HCWs' biomedical training is meant to have prepared them to deal objectively with all illnesses. Their training legitimizes their position as expert and extends authority and power to them. HCWs are expected to be among those whom Goffman

(1963: 41) has called "the wise": people "whose special situation has made them intimately privy to the life of the stigmatized individual and sympathetic with it." To some degree, then, idealized expectations regarding post-disclosure acceptance like those held for family and friends may be extended to HCWs by PHAs.

Notwithstanding health policy and practice are deeply embedded in general cultural values and consequently medical models and attitudes reflect lay values, beliefs and attitudes (Scambler 1984; Loustaunau and Sobo 1997). HCWs themselves share societal norms and attitudes. There is evidence that HCWs may have limited understanding about the psychological and social complexities of many conditions (e.g. dwarfism; see Ablon 1981), and social interactions between 'normal' HCWs and patients 'spoiled' by stigmatizing illness may be as marked by social disruption as they are in other settings.

Yet social interaction with HCWs is critical in mediating the social impact a stigmatizing disease has on a patient's social adjustment to being associated with a discreditable disease. Especially because they are seen as 'experts', and supposed to be so 'wise', negative reactions or tactless comments from HCWs are a potential source of trauma for those they serve, and can often be more damaging than the conditions themselves. For example, the most traumatic aspects of the birth and development of dwarf children may be related to doctors' ill-advised statements to the family (Ablon 1981). People with epilepsy have reported that a doctor's diagnosis and pronouncement on the disease "made them into epileptics" (Scambler 1984: 213). HCWs thus not only treat the physical manifestations of disease but also shape the social adaptation of patients. This is a task for which they are given very limited formal training.

HCW attitudes to PHAs

Numerous studies examine the knowledge and behaviour of HCWs with regard to treating PHAs. Hospital physicians, nurses and social workers in Chicago (Dworkin et al. 1991), general practitioners or GPs in Marseilles (Morin et al. 1995), dental and medical students in Pittsburgh (Weyant et al. 1994), physicians, nurses and technologists in Ontario (Taerk et al. 1993), undertakers in London's East End (Howarth 1993) and many others have expressed concerns to researchers. Studies consistently show that a major barrier to HCWs' treatment of PHAs is fear of infection. This seems to have a greater effect than homophobia, dislike of IDUs, the cost of treating seropositive people, or the terminal nature of AIDS (Taerk et al. 1993; Weyant et al. 1994; Dworkin et al. 1991; Ross and Hunter 1991). Notwithstanding, and as noted in Chapter 2, the fear of infection does not necessarily reflect the threat of infection and may be exaggerated due to the stigma of AIDS.

HCWs' fear of infection is largely related to the procedures involved in the care of PHAs, and HCWs who practise the most invasive procedures report the highest level of concern (Dworkin *et al.* 1991; Weyant *et al.* 1994; Ross and Hunter 1991). Level of fear is thus context-dependent, and perception of risk is related to actual risk. But prejudices interact with real transmission threats in complex ways, as we show below (and see Chapter 2). For example, take the fact that familiarity with a practice makes it more routine and it is thus less likely to be considered risky (see Chapter 3; see also Rhodes 1995). Thus, HCWs who spend the most time treating PHAs and therefore have a higher actual risk tend to have a diminished perception of risk (Kunzel and Sadowsky 1993) and less fear of infection (Gallop *et al.* 1991).

Studies of HCWs tend to be cross-sectional, making it difficult to assess changes over time. However, the more recent literature reports less fear from HCWs and the issuing of standard guidelines (e.g. by the Hospital Infection Society and the Surgical Infection Study Group 1992) has doubtless led to more routinization of practice and less stigmatizing behaviour. It is therefore likely that stigmatizing reactions to, and unprofessional behaviour toward, PHAs have decreased over time.

Stigmatization stories

In the literature, PHAs and their informal carers report many instances of stigmatization from HCWs, such as a doctor who, without his patient's knowledge or consent, wrote to "warn [her] employers" (anon 1992), or being made to use a separate hospital toilet with "control of infection" posted on it (Richardson and Boll 1992). Such experiences, or even just tales of them, may deter PHAs from seeking health care.

Gay PHAs in London, for example, have been found reluctant to register or consult with a GP (Wadsworth and McCann 1992). Many specialist units for PHAs have arisen largely to help PHAs avoid stigmatizing HCW behaviour, which they fear will occur in general practices. Satisfaction among patients utilizing specialist units tends to be high (e.g. Robinson and Croucher 1994; see also Cleary *et al.* 1992). There is concern, however, that specialist units are themselves stigmatized and that this may deter PHAs from attending.

HCWs and PHAs in Scotland

Participants at all sites had stories to tell about poor treatment or stigmatizing health-care events (although we heard some stories about wonderful care too). The Scottish research specifically examined how stigma affects the relationship between PHAs and HCWs in health care settings, and the findings discussed in the sections below come from the Scottish data set.[2]

Satisfaction ratings

A section on health care was included in the Scottish interviews described in Chapter 4. We asked participants about in-patient, out-patient, GP, and dental experiences and contacts with health visitors. We asked how satisfied they had been with the care and whether they had experienced any problems with any aspect of treatment.

In the course of annual interviews (n = 66), in response to questions about problems they had encountered in health care settings since being diagnosed HIV positive, 127 specific causes of dissatisfaction were reported by 47 people. In the second interview (n = 40)[3] a location question was added in order to compare satis-faction across treatment sites. Participants reported dissatisfaction with about one-third of hospitals where they had attended as in-patients, about one-sixth of out-patient departments, and about one-quarter of the GPs and dentists they had consulted. Dissatisfaction with health visitors was much lower: less than one-twelfth of health visitors who had been consulted.

Scrutiny of the data suggests that those who had been diagnosed longest reported the most stigmatizing incidents. This might be due to the fact that they had had more contact with HCWs over the course of their illness, or because they had acquired greater familiarity with hospitals and therefore had greater confid-ence to complain when they were dissatisfied. However, those with an AIDS diagnosis, particularly those nearing death, tended to be very complimentary about their care.

Some dissatisfactions were not specifically related to HIV, but were the kind of complaints commonly expressed by health care consumers: lack of continuity of care, being seen by junior doctors working on six-month rotation, having to wait despite having a fixed appointment. Some of the IDUs reported arguing with physicians about the level of methadone prescribed; this may have happened without HIV. And some dissatisfaction might have been related to a general mistrust of the health care system; for example, there was some explicit concern, especially among those offered AZT or newer drug therapies, that they were being used as "guinea pigs."

Ninety-two (72%) of the 127 specific incidents cited were directly related to the stigma of HIV.[4] Incidents relating to HCWs fear of treating PHAs were most prevalent. Next were problems related to the double stigma of HIV and the subsequent stigmatization of all PHAs and places where they are treated. A third important category related to confidentiality. Each type of complaint is found in the accounts of members of all transmission groups and in relation to all health care settings, although some variation was noted (more of which in Chapter 11).

Fear of contagion

Participants reported many incidents where, fearing infection, HCWs tried to avoid body contact, either by refusing to treat them adequately, or by wearing what was seen as too much protective clothing. Some participants also reported being placed in physical isolation which prevented them having contact with other patients.

Refusal to treat adequately

Two participants (both prisoners) reported that non-essential surgical operations were cancelled after HCWs were informed by prison medical staff they were HIV positive, and six participants reported being refused treatment by a GP and seven by a dentist. All these refusals were believed by participants to be HIV-related.

Refusals to treat were often subtle as, for example, when a GP insisted a participant who moved to a house that was farther away sign up with a practice nearer to her new home. Many community dentists routinely referred participants to hospital dental departments after disclosure of HIV status. These kinds of refusals were usually relatively polite. Occasionally, however, brutal rejection was reported. Annie, an ex-IDU and recovering alcoholic who was trying to find a GP, had this to say:

> Well I needed a doctor because I had moved into the area and I went down to the doctor's surgery and I asked if I could become a patient and the lady started to hand me, you know, like a form to fill in and I says to her, "Oh I'm HIV positive," and she says "Oh I don't know if Doctor will see you but take a seat." So I sat down beside the rest of the patients and

> this doctor comes just right across to me, got me by here, the collar, and
> he says to me, "You'll have to leave the surgery."

As distressing as this story is, our experience with this participant reminds us that we need to adopt a critical approach to participants' accounts. Annie was reporting an incident retrospectively. She made no mention of whether or not she had been using drugs or alcohol at the time, nor whether she had been a previous patient at this GP's surgery when she was using drugs.[5] Participants' natural desire to manage their presentations of self needs to be considered when evaluating the self-reports we quote from. The quotes remain, however, verbatim accounts of the perceptions of PHAs; the very fact that seropositivity takes the blame for so many negative occurrences is one of the main points of our discussion of identity and HIV. The social context in which HIV becomes blameworthy is very real and can be very threatening.

Another example of reluctance to treat in seen in this report from Thomas, who disclosed his HIV status to the doctor on duty when seeking emergency treatment for an ear infection.

> He did not want to touch me after that. He just said, "I am writing you a
> prescription for antibiotics. Go to the Infectious Diseases Hospital or your
> own doctor. I don't want anything to do with you because I don't know
> anything about HIV." I said "I am not here about HIV I am here about my
> ears."

Participants frequently reported HCWs' fear of touching them or their bodily fluids, and three respondents were left overnight in fluid-soaked bedclothes. Heather was forced to sleep in sheets "all covered in blood" after she gave birth. Brian, a prisoner who had a similar experience when he had had teeth extracted in a general hospital, remarked, "I have never been so glad to get back to prison in my life." Whether people without HIV being treated in those surgeries would be left with bloody sheets or towels is unclear; nonetheless, the perception that this was due to HIV was overwhelming.

Barrier protection

Fear of infection was most dramatically illustrated by participants' reports of receiving treatment from HCWs "dressed like spacemen." Twenty-one individuals cited incidents involving HCWs either wearing what was seen to be an unnecessary

125

amount of protective clothing or for their insensitivity in letting patients see them in such clothing.

HCWs wearing so-called "space suits" were most often reported where there was a high risk of body contact with participant's bodily fluids.

Betty: I've been in the jail to a dentist and he was like a spaceman. That was before I got all my teeth out. He was all – all you could see were his eyes through a wee plastic, like a wee windscreen thing and it was all big boots and – but that was years ago.

Gina: They had on like these big masks, they had like big space suits on and I was just thinking you know this is all because I'm HIV positive and they must be terrified of me. ...I didn't agree with the treatment I had got. OK if they want to take precautions fine but why don't they put you to sleep before letting me actually see that.

While many dentists and other clinicians today wear protective goggles or face masks and other gear on a routine basis, many (especially in the UK) did not in the early 90s, when these data were collected. Participants often reported that the use of protective clothing was unnecessary. Many also reported instances of over-dressing where there was no risk of infection. For instance, Vicky said, "When I went to the dentist there was this frigging nurse, she never came anywhere near me and was all gowned up. She wasn't even treating me and she was wearing two pairs of gloves and wellingtons [rubber boots]."

Participants were aware that during some medical procedures there was a small risk of HIV transmission and they were concerned that HCWs should take reasonable precautions. While overdoing it was frowned upon, sometimes participants expressed concern that HCWs did not protect themselves sufficiently. Two participants, for example, reported disclosing when a HCW started to take blood or examine their teeth without gloves on. Their stories about these incidents reflected ideas about others' need to know and one's moral responsibility to protect others from infection.

Reasons for HCW fear

Participants pointed to HCWs' fear of infection as the principal source of stigma in health care settings. In this respect, the views of PHAs in this study were in concordance with the attitudes of HCWs as described in the literature cited above. Nonetheless, in a number of reported instances, the level of fear appeared to be unrelated to the actual risk (recall the dental nurse in wellingtons [rubber boots]). Such incidents tended to occur in settings where HCWs were not familiar with HIV. Fear seemed greatest in non-specialist units, such as general hospitals.

It is not surprising that interactions between PHAs and HCWs unfamiliar with HIV are strained, uncomfortable and tense, as social disruption is part of the process and product of stigmatization (see Goffman 1963; Albrecht *et al.* 1982). Continued contact, however, tends to reduce the salience of an abnormal characteristic by a process of "normalisation" (Davis 1964); the stigmatized individual is eventually accepted as 'normal', or at least ascribed an identity based on the person and not the stigmatizing characteristic. HCWs who have regular contact with PHAs over time are likely to achieve normalized interactions and these individuals (e.g. HCWs in specialist HIV units) were most frequently praised by our participants.

HCW fears disproportionate to actual risk were probably based less upon ignorance about HIV transmission than upon the dirty and dangerous image associated with AIDS. This may explain why fear tended to be greater in procedures involving symbolically important areas of the body – socially salient areas, such as the mouth and throat, used for conversation, or the vagina, used for sex and childbearing (*cf.* Sobo 1993b). Research linking fear of contagion with the reality of transmission risks should take into account the disproportionate degree of fear associated with socially significant body parts; the threat of contagion is not a uniformly relevant fear. This supports findings in Kunzel and Sadowsky (1993) and Gallop *et al.* (1991) that the contexts that generate the most fear are not those in which it is most statistically justifiable. It may also explain why, although all HCWs were no doubt aware that one does not 'catch' HIV through skin-to-skin contact, touch of the stigmatized person was nevertheless tainted by his or her deeply discrediting attribute.

Notwithstanding that much HCW fear is related to a real, albeit low, risk of transmission (e.g. through a needle stick injury), HCW fear does not appear to equate directly with actual risk. The calculus is more complex, which explains why HCW fear may occasionally be entirely unrelated to the actual risk of transmission. Rather than examining the actual risks entailed in performing surgery, taking blood, changing bed linen or filing notes, some HCWs may view each contact with PHAs, regardless of what is involved, as risky. Thus, whilst the metaphorical otherness of PHAs and the social threat that they represented may have prompted the use of space suits by HCWs in low or no-risk situations, so too may PHA's otherness have generated actual fears of contracting HIV amongst the HCWs with whom they came into contact.[6]

Routes of transmission

HCWs' often unwarranted fear of contagion heightened the social risk for many PHAs. Another source was the common HCW assumption that all PHAs are gay or use drugs; because of this, participants said, they were treated badly. Cathy, who had never used drugs, said that HCWs "just presumed things ... and automatically thought I was a drug user." Said Gina, a heterosexual infected by her partner, "Being taken to the operating theatre [room] was horrible because one of the doctors said, 'Oh, you're the junkie aren't you.' ...I remember falling asleep but crying and kind of saying you know, 'No I'm not, I'm not'."

Thomas, an ex-IDU for many years, complained that he was never able to shake the drug-using image in his interactions with HCWs, who seemed to expect bad behaviour from him. Many of the IDUs complained that they were not given enough pain-killing medicine because, as Mitch explained, HCWs thought they were "looking for a free stone [drug-induced high]"; consequently, sometimes they had to endure severe pain. Negative reactions related to homosexuality, real or imputed, were less often reported than those related to IDUs.

Specialist treatment centres

To counteract stigma experienced in general health care settings, a number of treatment centres were set up in Scotland specifically for PHAs. Participants generally spoke warmly about these, portraying them as "a good thing," as the social risk of attending them was low. Paul argued that specialist units offer "people secure space and in some ways if you're in a specialist unit at least you're going to feel OK about it rather than hiding in your room, you know, frightened to come out."

This opinion was not shared by all participants. Those who reported that they had not been infected through gay sex or injecting drugs often held negative attitudes toward those who were. They tended to associate HIV centres with gays and IDUs and therefore saw them as more socially risky spaces than general healthcare settings. Derek, a heterosexual, said he "hated the stigma" attached to being a patient at the HIV clinic. He attended sessions aimed toward IDUs to minimize the possibility of being recognized. James, a haemophiliac, complained that at the specialist centre "there's druggies all over the place," and most people with haemophilia expressed a preference for receiving HIV treatment at the general hospital where they were already enrolled for their blood disorder.

Keeping secrets

An inevitable consequence of the heightened social risk of being HIV positive is concern about confidentiality. Although the majority of participants were satisfied with confidentiality procedures, one-fifth of those who had been in-patients were not, and a number of confidentiality breaches were reported also for out-patient clinics, GP and dental surgeries. For example, David's dentist disclosed his HIV status to a mutual friend without permission; Mitch's GP told his mother, without even informing him that he had done so.

Most confidentiality breaches were less blatant. Some participants saw them as inevitable, and attributable to informal information networks among HCWs (*cf.* Huby 1999). Because of these networks, several participants described confidentiality as "a joke." Although they were mostly able to rationalize that HCWs needed to share information about them to improve care, participants often felt that HCWs "bandy information about" carelessly. Said Bob, "They don't seem to treat it in a serious manner, it's just another bit of useless information that they've been given. That's the impression that one gets and as I say, it doesn't help when your files go missing between departments."

Hospital files were a major problem for in-patients, who felt they were not sufficiently protected. There was concern that anyone in the hospital could read a file and one man said he "caught an auxiliary" [a health care assistant] reading his. Another said that when he was in hospital his file was "lying on a desk with a big sticker saying 'HIV positive' on it. Anybody could have walked past and lifted it up."

The lack of privacy in hospital wards also was problematic. Although some participants complained about feeling stigmatized when put in a private room, there were also drawbacks to a general ward. For example, when Keith was in hospital following a haemophilia bleed, he felt concerned that the patient in the neighbouring bed would realize his HIV status when the nurse reminded him in a loud voice to take his AZT.

Gary, who had previously worked in the health care system, said:

> I can remember when I was diagnosed and I knew a member of the staff up there, I'd known him for some time, we'd worked together, and I felt very unsure at the time and I really didn't want him to know. So I said to the counsellor "I really don't want him to know," and she said, "Well we have regular team meetings where, you know, new cases are discussed." And I said, "Well I don't want you to mention my name at the team meeting," and she said, "Oh but we always do that," and I said, "But I

forbid you to do that." And she was quite shocked at that because there is an assumption in professional circles that you can pass on information willy-nilly, and I don't think that's proper.

Gary's story illustrates the confidentiality challenge faced by PHAs receiving treatment in small communities. Jim, a gay man who lived in a small town, switched himself to a general practice in another town as although he did not "doubt their confidentiality ... things do slip now and again."

Even in a large town, network membership can endanger confidentiality. Glasgow and Edinburgh, the cities where most of the Scottish participants resided, both have sizeable populations but the gay and drug-using communities in both are not large and a number of participants reported seeing people they knew while seeking care. This rarely caused a great deal of anxiety – in at least two cases it was the basis for deeper friendship – but it did make people uneasy about confidentiality, and it did add to the socially risky nature of health care settings.

The impact of stigmatization by HCWs

Stigmatizing incidents generally aroused anger, indignation and hurt. Donald claimed to have "suffered far more mental strain and humiliation in hospital than physical pain." The humour that accompanied many participants' reports of painful incidents indexed the emotive reaction they unleashed. That is, in order to cope psychologically with stigmatizing incidents many participants made light of them or challenged them by making fun of the HCWs. Likewise, frequent use of the term 'spaceman' to describe HCWs evoked the somewhat surreal nature of the incidents.

Frequent use of the term 'spaceman' also suggests social learning as stories and expressions circulate amongst PHAs. This colours perceptions as well as narrations; shared understandings about what might happen or what has happened to others alters the landscape of risk, increasing felt stigma.

Notwithstanding, enacted stigmatization in health care settings had a very negative impact upon many participants. Total avoidance of health care was reported rarely but Donald in retrospect said that he wished he "had stayed at home." In general, participants felt they had to take advantage of the health care offered to them despite the threat of stigmatization so that they might maintain their health for as long as possible.

All but three of 40 Scottish participants followed-up after one year were registered with a doctor and in all but one case the doctor was aware of their HIV status. They also received out-patient treatment from specialist clinics but many reported that they found the HIV clinic "a constant reminder" of their condition, and so chose to attend at infrequent, irregular intervals. Similarly, dental care tended to be limited (by those who generally did visit dentists prior to diagnosis) to absolutely necessary treatment rather than routine visits. One man had stopped going completely as he did not wish to disclose his serostatus to his dentist, a thing he felt he had to do to continue to receive treatment.

In many health care settings, participants' serostatus was known prior to consultation, largely as a result of the informal HCW information network whereby clinic consultants would inform patients' GPs or vice-versa (*cf.* Huby 1999). This was usually with the patient's consent. The information web did not normally extend to hospital departments to which patients referred themselves, such as Accident and Emergency departments, or to community dental practices. In such settings, participants had to decide whether or not to disclose and six of the 40 described instances where they had not disclosed during treatment for fear of a negative reaction.[7] Said Stuart:

> What I really wanted was decent teeth. The dentist I go to ... he doesn't know I am a haemophiliac and he doesn't know I am HIV, but he wears gloves. ...[Disclosing] would make it all too complicated ... I would not get the job done the way I have got it done. I tried for two years to get it done at the hospital and it is two years that I have wasted. My teeth just deteriorated.

Some participants, aware that some PHAs do not disclose and that many more people are not aware of their status, having never been tested, felt they had been dealt with unfairly when they received stigmatizing treatment after disclosure. Tony disclosed his HIV status to his dentist and as a result he was asked always to attend for treatment at the last appointment of the day. He complained, "I may have not known. I may have decided not to tell them, so it is ridiculous" that the practice reacted this way.

PHAs receiving treatment have, to some extent, placed trust in HCWs to maximize the quality and quantity of their lives. Negative reactions can erode any such trust, leading PHAs to shun health care settings at the cost of their health.

More than physical health can be damaged. Relations with HCWs are very important for the adjustment of people with stigmatized illnesses, particularly those that are concealed and generally not disclosed to others. HCWs may be among the few people who know about a person's serostatus and a negative reaction may lead to negative identity formation through an internalization of attributed danger and spoilage. Recall Gina's conclusion upon seeing HCWs dressed in space suits: "They must be terrified of me." This was confirmation, to her, of her terrifying identity.

Social risk in public settings

There is clear evidence that the Scottish PHAs encountered what they felt to be fear and loathing from HCWs. Indeed, the level of dissatisfaction expressed is considerably greater than that reported in most satisfaction-with-care studies; these tend to generate generally approving answers (Williams 1994). It is, however, important to qualify the findings in a number of ways. First, participants may have been overly focused upon negative experiences, as they were asked about difficulties and problems. And the data did contain contradictions. For example, eight participants reported that psychosocial support offered by counselling services was inadequate while seven singled this out for praise. And while some GPs were criticized for lack of knowledge or for complaining about the cost of certain treatments, more often they were praised by participants for their caring attitude or their willingness to learn and for "doing their best." Many participants felt that they had established positive relationships with particular HCWs over time. In fact, most participants were satisfied most of the time with the health care that they received and had very few complaints despite receiving treatment for several years; 19 of 66 had no complaints whatsoever. Specialist units such as hospices and respite care centres, specialist HIV-hospital wards, and outpatient clinics were singled out for particular praise.

Another important consideration is that the incidents reported occurred in or prior to the early 1990s, when the data were collected. The most florid examples of stigmatization mostly occurred in the more distant past. Participants themselves reported that things had improved and many ended their recountings with the caveat, "but that was a long time ago." Nevertheless, some of the reports of stigma were among the newly diagnosed. And similar stories were recounted by more recently interviewed participants, in the New Mexico and North-East England samples. Stigmatization in health care settings remains a concern of PHAs and professional bodies of HCWs (see Horsman and Sheeran 1995).

It is clear that health care settings are perceived as socially risky by PHAs and there is some evidence to support this assessment. In health care settings, non-disclosure is not usually an option. Notions related to kinship and friendship do not surface as motivating factors; instead, it is the instrumental relationship between HCW and PHA that underlies disclosure. Unlike other socially distant people with whom one has no inherently expressive ties, HCWs are supposed to know about one's health, especially if they are called on in relation to HIV's effects. Further, they are understood as experts on medical issues, and expected to be wise or well-informed and unbiased in regard to diseases, including AIDS. Interactions with HCWs are thus vital in shaping PHAs self-constructions and their management of the "stigma trajectory" (Alonzo and Reynolds 1995) that unfolds during the course of the disease.

In some of the incidents described above, the participant's HIV status seems to have achieved "master status" (Hughes 1945: 303); seropositivity becomes the summary of the individual; the HCW treats the seropositive and not the person. Such objectification can only reinforce the growth of the seropositive aspect of identity at the expense of other components of self, and so can stymie more well-rounded personhood.

Interactions with HCWs provide further evidence of the 'double stigma' of HIV. Even participants who had not been infected sexually or through injecting drugs reported being deemed gay or an IDU, and many felt they were stigmatized because of the association. The double stigma of HIV affects all PHAs, however they are infected, and this can make HIV-related stigma more acute for PHAs who are neither gay nor drug injectors as well as for those who are not 'out' about being so. People with haemophilia, those infected heterosexually, and those who are drug users or gay but not well adjusted to that fact (Lang 1991) may be particularly vulnerable to developing a sense of self-loathing after stigmatizing incidents. To use Crawford's (1994) terminology, these PHAs may experience a breakdown of the boundary between self and other in that the 'stigmatizing self' who holds pejorative views about gay sex or drug use or PHAs is prompted by stigmatizing incidents to look in the mirror and self-identify as the 'unhealthy other'. This process may lead to a fractured identity. On the other hand, these PHAs may become (more) homophobic or anti-drug as they try to reaffirm their place in society and their claims to moral personhood.

The impact of personally experienced stigmatizing interactions with HCWs (of which there were a substantial number) notwithstanding, the degree to which one's internalized unhealthy otherness depends on them is unclear. Further, whereas a PHA may have felt that protective clothing worn by an HCW was excessive and may have perceived an HCW's attitude as moralistic, it could be that the HCW was taking sensible precautions. And avoidance of health care to avoid potential stigmatization, deciding not to disclose HIV status in health settings, or dislike of the attitude of some HCWs cannot be categorized as overt stigmatization. Rather, these actions and reactions emanate from a fear of stigmatization. They emanate from participants' internalisation of stigmatizing attitudes whereby they feel devalued as a result of their HIV status; that is, they reflect felt rather than enacted stigma.

Although this chapter has illustrated the social risks of the health care setting, in general PHAs spoke highly of HCWs and found their interactions with them beneficial. The data presented here and in the preceding chapters suggest that PHAs may overestimate the social risk of interaction with HCWs. It is our disheartening conclusion that an elevated sense of risk may inhibit some PHAs from seeking health care. An exaggerated sense of risk also may keep PHAs from fulfilling their conjugal ideals, as the next chapter shows.

Notes

1   Aboulafia (1998) estimates that there are approximately 5000 percutaneous exposures to blood known to be infected with HIV among health care workers in the US each year. The risk of transmission after percutaneous exposure has been estimated to be 0.3 per cent.
2   Much of this chapter is based, with kind permission, on Green and Platt (1997).
3   In year two, 26 individuals were lost to follow-up; see Chapter 4.
4   The distinction between stigmatizing and non-stigmatizing incidents was based on PHAs perception of them. Those that they clearly felt to be related to the stigma of HIV were classed as stigmatizing whereas those that they felt were not (even if they were related to HIV) were not.
5   Although in many cases we might have attempted to elicit such information, probing was inappropriate during this particular self-report.
6   Some HCWs may have over-dressed because they were truly afraid of contracting HIV. Due to the dramatic manner in which AIDS entered the public consciousness, the risk of transmission tends to be greatly exaggerated (e.g. Klepinger et al. 1993). Help lines set up after health professionals disclose their seropositivity attract thousands of calls from worried former patients (Ellis 1993), although the only recorded incident of a HCW infecting patients was that of a dentist in Florida who transmitted the virus to six identified patients (Scully and Mortimer 1994). It is likely that some HCWs, like members of the public, also exaggerate to some degree the risk of transmission from treating PHAs and are thereby overly fearful about caring for them.
7   The actual number of non-disclosure incidents was probably higher: the social taboo surrounding non-disclosure may have led to under-reporting.

Chapter 9

Disclosure in sexual settings: identifying the issues

Relationship type and disclosure dilemmas

The kind of relationship that a PHA has with a potential disclosee (employee–boss, father-son, sister-brother, spousal, etc.) is an important factor in the self-disclosure situation. We have seen that social distance plays a key mediating role here, as does whether the relationship's inaugural reason for being is HIV (as with health care workers or HCWs; see Chapter 8). We have also seen that others' reactions have great potential to affect the way in which a PHA incorporates or otherwise deals with the HIV-positive dimension of his or her identity.

As discussed in the previous chapter, HCWs are expected to 'know better'; negative reactions on their part can have profound impact. For reasons discussed in this chapter and illustrated with our findings in the next, the reactions of PHAs' lovers to news of their positive serostatus can be just as crucial as HCW reactions. Further, more profound social risks may be entailed: for example, disclosing to a lover may lead to the loss of that relationship. And a sexual partner might not honour one's confidentiality concerns – concerns generated and maintained in part by the stigma attached to HIV and its stereotypic (and stigmatized) modes of transmission. So while disclosure to sexual partners may seem to outsiders as imperative, the enormous social risks entailed may make it less than appealing to PHAs themselves.

Chances for transmission of HIV are much higher in the health care and sexual arenas than they are in arenas in which contact is purely social (e.g. with friends and non-spousal family members). Precautions taken by HCWs to minimize chances for infection can be justified not only by reference to actual risk levels but also because the relationship between HCW and PHA is understood as, at base, distant and instrumental. Precautions taken in the sexual arena are not so easily dealt with. Whilst HCWs should be able to deal objectively with HIV, which is, after all, the basis of the HCW-PHA relationship and, often, a chosen element in one's job description (McGarrahan 1994), HIV is not generally something one's sexual partner(s) expect to be told about.[1] Moreover, AIDS-related precautions are generally seen as out of place when sexual partners are in love: love brings people closer together on the social distance scale and, as we show in this chapter, safer sex generally is seen to contradict such closeness (*cf.* Sobo 1993a, 1995b).

Love (or: our cultural construction of it) is key. Love and related emotional expression has become a valued aspect of conjugality in modern Western society and part of a cultural theory of self-development according to which one's "unique self" can be attained through emotional intimacy in the private sphere (Cancian 1987: 27–28). As sex-role distinctions have diminished, people's capacity and desire for intimacy in the context of conjugal relations has increased. The private sphere or domestic realm has become the main arena for the expression of love and the emotional sharing this entails (regarding the ideological functions of this, see Rapp 1987). Research in the USA has shown that people conceptualize the intimacy or social closeness of lovers as built on self-disclosure, partner disclosure, and self- and partner responsiveness to such sharing of inner feelings and important secrets (Laurenceau *et al.* 1998; Cancian 1987). We have no reason to think love any different in the UK.

Social closeness equals emotional closeness. For this reason, social distance is not diminished merely because people have sex. Indeed, some people reserve certain kinds of sex for those who are most socially distant (Handwerker 1993).[2] Social distance persists with casual sexual relations, and honesty expectations for casual partners are generally much lower than those for primary partners, friends and family members. Thus a casual partner's 'need to know', as perceived by the PHA, may be minimal because of love's absence. And with love's absence, condom use is generally less problematic. Condom-related distancing and duplicity cannot be imputed when expectations for devotion and full disclosure are not present to begin with.

Nonetheless, and largely for cultural reasons, the sexual arena is one in which, and about which, emotions and thoughts are highly charged and vested. This makes the institution of safer sex or talk about one's serostatus very difficult indeed, whether with primary or casual partners. Disclosing to each type of partner involves different yet overlapping challenges, as we show in the next chapter. Here, we briefly examine previous research on the topic.

Malicious non-disclosure[3]

We have seen that there are many drawbacks to disclosing and that non-disclosure may be viewed as a rational choice made by a person trying to maintain a healthy social life. The media, however, often describes non-disclosure as if malicious. We also know that part of the process of coping with AIDS may involve anger (McCain and Gramling 1992). Fury and rage may turn a person rancorous and vindictive. When one feels a need to seek revenge but does not know against whom to seek it, any human target may do (and in the case of AIDS it is frequently difficult to track down the source of one's infection, should one desire to do so). But, generally, anger subsides and PHAs are content to fight AIDS, not other people (McCain and Gramling 1992).

Still, rumours of vindictive individuals spreading HIV among unknowing innocents, as described in Chapter 2, do circulate. Such rumours appeal to many because, faced with the uncontrollable likes of the AIDS pandemic, urges to attribute blame, scapegoat, and hunt out so-called witches run high (Sobo *et al.* 1997; *cf.* Farmer 1992).[4] People may feel defenceless against non-disclosers, as they often do against AIDS. Insinuating themselves into the lives of innocents, vindictive seropositive monsters work, metaphorically, just like HIV itself, which slips into the body unnoticed and for which there is no cure or escape once one's cells have been tricked into reproducing it.

All states in the USA have laws regarding seropositivity disclosure but purposeful non-disclosure is a shadowy area, legally. A move to criminalize intentional HIV transmission began in the early 1990s. By 1993, 25 US states had criminal transmission laws on the books (*Nation's Health* 1993). In the UK, no laws have been passed yet but there have been calls to criminalize "murderous intent" on the part of PHAs.

While most agree that intentionally inflicting harm and conspiring to murder (albeit slowly and tortuously, as would be the case with AIDS) is wrong, criminalization may not be wise. Criminal transmission laws may be used in selective scapegoating; in the USA, such laws are commonly used against prostitutes and prisoners (*Nation's Health* 1993). Moreover, intentions are particularly hard to discern when the sexual arena serves as the site of transmission. The emotions surrounding sexual events (especially taboo ones) often run high and there is a very real danger that people with vendettas, such as spurned ex-lovers, will vengefully incriminate targeted PHAs.

Self-disclosure research

Is non-disclosure to sexual partners as malicious as the rhetoric supporting criminalization suggests it is? Do actual disclosure rates support a fear of non-disclosure? In the early 1990s, when we began our studies, much of what we knew about self-disclosure specifically to lovers came from studies examining the efficacy of partner notification or third-party disclosure programmes. These programmes, through which third parties such as public health officials notify PHAs' partners, free PHAs from the burden of having to share their news.

Some research indicates that third-party disclosure is successful if measured in economic terms (i.e. averting infections that would cost more money to treat).[5] In addition, partner notification programmes offer a way to identify the possibility of infection in people (partners and ex-partners) who might not otherwise suspect it (*Lancet* 1991). Giesecke *et al.* (1991) argue that partner notification programmes can be more effective at identifying HIV-positive individuals than large-scale screening efforts (people who do not see themselves as at risk may not seek testing; see Sobo 1994). Notification programmes also might be more effective than self-disclosure, at least in relation to the notification of previous or casual partners.[6]

But what about self-disclosure in current sexual relations? Many HIV-infected individuals are not aware of their serostatus. But others are, and serostatus disclosure can affect the risk-related decisions that they and their sexual partners make.

Research focused specifically on sexuality among HIV-positive people has been very hard to come by. Ross's (1995) edited volume was among the first to attempt to fill the gap. There has been a growing trend to investigate sexual behaviour among PHAs, especially gay male PHAs, with the express aim of using findings to stem transmission. But to our knowledge the first organized attempt to publish on this topic did not come until 1998, when a special issue of a US AIDS journal focused on so-called 'risk behaviour' was released (Kalichman and Fisher 1998). As the editors of that special issue note,

> Much too little is known about the dynamics of risk [for the seropositive].
> ...Since only people with HIV can transmit HIV, the lack of such work is

very surprising and disturbing. ...In a very real sense, we have missed some of the most critical targets for research and intervention (p. 87).

Most PHA 'risk behaviour' studies are quantitatively oriented and data regarding the sociocultural contexts in which risks are taken are thin. Further, while risk to one's partner's physical health and, in some cases, to one's own (e.g. through cross-infection) is considered; the *social* risks of *not* participating in unprotected sex are rarely acknowledged. Finally, despite attentiveness to differences in participants' 'risk-taking' (unsafe sex) rates according to serostatus, knowledge of serostatus, time since diagnosis, and the like, most seropositive risk-taking studies do not include self-disclosure or even one's partner's knowledge of one's serostatus as a research variable.

The lack of attention to self-disclosure is nothing new. Few publications discussing self-disclosure were available when our research began – although many had mentioned the topic in passing. For example, McKeganey and Barnard (1992) devoted a few pages of their book on IDUs to a few participants' comments on the issue. McKeganey and Barnard sought to illuminate what it was like to be HIV positive and to show that PHAs and IDUs in general were neither abnormal nor dangerous. But most other authors' references to self-disclosure to partners are less considered. For example, in concluding their report on risk reduction among HIV-positive women, Kline and VanLandingham mentioned that "anecdotal evidence suggests that in several cases women failed to disclose their serostatus to their partners" (1994: 401). The problematic use of the concept "failure" in relation to non-disclosure notwithstanding, the extent of non-disclosure and its effects on risk reduction were left unexamined.[7]

Pivnick (1993) also touched on non-disclosure to partners. Although Pivnick's main concern was the meaning of condoms among women attending a methadone clinic, she noted that 14 of the 16 married seropositive women in her sample had disclosed their serostatus to their partners. The two who had not self-disclosed insisted that their partners use condoms with them but, rather than telling their partners that this was because of HIV, they said that the condoms were for contraception (pp. 436–438; such diversionary tactics are explored in Chapter 10).

As Table 9.1 shows, the proportion of women who self-disclosed is quite similar to the proportion of self-disclosers to primary partners found in research publications specifically concerned with self-disclosure to sexual partners – little of which until recently existed, and most of which focuses on gay or bisexual men. For instance, using data from mostly white homo- and bisexual men recruited in Dallas (TX), Denver (CO), Seattle (WA), and Long Beach (CA), Schnell *et al.* (1992) found a

Table 9.1 Serostatus self-disclosure frequencies[1]

	To primary partners	To secondary partners
Hays et al. (1993)	98%	
Mansergh et al. (1995)	86% – 93%	
Marks et al. (1992a)	69%	36%
Perry et al. (1994)	77%	42% – 47%
Pivnick (1993)	88%	
Schnell et al. (1992)	89%	
Stein et al. (1998)	88%	
Wolitski et al. (1998)	89%	34%

1 Study methods differed; frequencies are not directly comparable

self-disclosure-to-partners rate of 89 per cent. Similarly, in their study of mostly white, mostly educated, mostly well-off homosexual San Francisco men, Hays et al. (1993) found that nearly all (98%) told their primary partners of their conditions; asymptomatic men were less likely than symptomatic men were to disclose their HIV status. Again, working with men, but this time with a multiethnic sample, Mansergh et al. (1995) found the same: participants reported self-disclosure rates of 86 and 93 per cent, the former for asymptomatic PHAs and the latter for those with symptoms.

Marks et al. carried out research with lower income men from Los Angeles, most of whom were Hispanic and homo- or bisexual (1992a, 1992b, 1991). Subjects favoured self-disclosure to partners known as seropositive (1991: 1322; regarding the impact that a potential disclosee's sexual orientation has on self-disclosure see Hays et al. 1993). Moreover, the likelihood of self-disclosure decreased as the number of partners in the previous year increased. About one in three (36%) men with two to four partners self-disclosed, while more than two in three (69%) men with one partner had (Marks et al. 1992a).

Another study, carried out by Perry et al. (1994; see also 1990b) with mostly white homosexual men of mixed incomes found a negative correlation between self disclosure to partners and perceived social support, having a spouse or live-in partner, and comfort about one's homosexual orientation. After a mean of just over two (2.3) years since initial notification of seropositive status, 86 per cent of the participants had informed at least one sex partner, present or past, primary or casual.[8] Participants were more likely to have informed primary sex partners, past or present (77 per cent had done so), than they were to have informed casual partners, past (47 per cent had done so) or present (42 per cent had done so). Fourteen per cent of the participants did not self-disclose to any partner at all.

More recently, Wolitski et al. (1998) reported a self disclosure to primary partners rate of 89 per cent. The rate for disclosing to casual partners was 34 per cent. The participants in Wolitski *et al.* were gay and bisexual men, and mostly white. In a similarly recent study conducted at two urban hospitals with an ethnically diverse sample of women and men, Stein *et al.* (1998) found that participants with one partner over the six months prior to the study were more than three times as likely to self-disclose to that partner than people with multiple partners. Eighty-eight per cent of the 99 participants with primary partners self-disclosed. This rate is similar to those seen among the samples of gay and bisexual men previously discussed.

In summary, as Table 9.1 shows, data from the early-mid 1990s suggested – and more recent work confirms – that the majority of PHAs tell their primary partners about their HIV status. But not all will do so and, moreover, most do not tell past or secondary partners about their health conditions. For example, Fisher *et al.* (1998) report that while 60 per cent of their participants (all men who have sex with men, less than half of whom had primary partners) had discussed their antibody status with known[9] partners in the past and would do so in the future, 34 per cent had not and never intended to discuss their serostatus with anonymous partners. Social distance calculations do seem to come into play as PHAs consider sexual partners' need to know.

Whether a partner is primary or casual, known or anonymous, non-disclosure undercuts his or her efforts to make informed decisions regarding safer sex. As Shtarkshall and Awerbuch point out, "Were the aware [seropositive] partner to disclose the relevant information, the unaware partner would be able to use the knowledge to assess his/her real risk of becoming infected" (1992: 124). Given the right conditions, the newly aware partner might approach sex more cautiously. Of course, people cannot actually compute their "real" risk levels; the calculations are far too complex. Even so, Shtarkshall and Awerbuch suggest that non-awareness of partner seropositivity correlates with people's underestimation of their AIDS risk levels.

The next chapter examines the strategies PHAs in our own research had for sharing serostatus information with their partners. As we will show, self-disclosure is a highly risky social gambit and one that is influenced heavily by the cultural expectations we hold in regard to our partners and our relationships with them.

Notes

1   Sobo's findings suggest that some PHAs' partners may actively work against disclosure. Some may choose to deny or ignore the possibility of a partners' positive serostatus in order to avoid confronting painful 'home truths' about the nature of their relationship or

    having to alter preferred patterns of interaction. Some examples are provided in Chapter 10 (regarding 'denial' amongst untested and seronegative women, see Sobo 1995b).

2 Handwerker (1993) has shown that men in Barbados prefer to have anal or other non-face-to-face sex with prostitutes. To have such sex with primary partners would, the men felt, be inappropriate and insulting to them.

3 With kind permission of the publishers, portions of Sobo (1995b, 1997) have been drawn on to frame the remaining sections in this chapter.

4 Whole groups have been faulted by some for originating the pandemic. Some blame Africans or Haitians; others blame the CIA or white supremacists for 'The AIDS Conspiracy' (Dalton 1989; Farmer 1992; Quimby 1992; Sobo *et al.* 1997; Turner 1993). Malicious non-disclosure by an individual differs little from a conspiratorial plot except that an individual rather than a highly-organized group lies lurking, ready to entrap.

5 In a study of CDC-funded counselling, testing, referral, and partner notification (CTRPN) programmes, Holtgrave *et al.* (1993) found that despite the fact that HIV's long incubation period can make identifying and locating exposed individuals extremely difficult, "for every 100 HIV-seropositive persons identified and reached by CTRPN services, at least 20 new HIV infections are averted" (p. 1225). Based on treatment cost calculations, "the CDC's expenditure on HIV CTRPN services results in a substantial net economic benefit to society" (p. 1229).

6 To test this, Landis *et al.* (1992) carried out a study in which mostly male, mostly Black, and mostly homo- or bisexual PHAs were randomly assigned to either a 'patient-referral group' – a group in which participants were made responsible for informing their partners of their seropositivity – or a 'provider-referral group' – a group in which a study counsellor notified the partners. The partners to be notified included all people with whom each study participant had had sex during the previous year. While the 'provider-referral group' succeeded in notifying fifty per cent of the partners, members of the 'patient-referral group' only notified seven per cent. Landis and colleagues concluded that leaving notification up to PHAs is 'quite ineffective' (p. 101).

7 One of the earliest publications regarding self-disclosure *per se* reported that a 'sizeable minority' of homo- and bisexual men did not plan to share positive test results with sexual partners (Kegeles *et al.* 1988). However, this publication reported only on *intentions* to communicate test results.

8 Seventy-one per cent of the participants had informed at least one present partner, and 70 per cent had informed at least one past partner.

9 In this research, known partners did include casual partners as well as primary partners.

Chapter 10

Reported reactions in sexual settings: our findings

In order to gain a clearer picture of the experiences PHAs have when their sexual partners know that they are infected with HIV, or when deciding if this should be the case, we collected data on self-disclosure and sexual relationships. This was the main focus of the research in New Mexico and formed the main starting point for the identity construction research in North-East England. We examine data from both sites in turn in this chapter, and look to the Scottish data for comparison where appropriate. We quote the participants liberally and, when appropriate, focus-group discourse is presented as conversation in order to preserve vital contextual information and to convey the key dimensions of the intersubjective debates carried on.

Disclosure to sexual partners in New Mexico[1]

In New Mexico, discussions and interviews wove back and forth around the same basic topics introduced in Chapters 6 and 7. Participants were especially concerned with a disclosee's need to know, and one's obligation to protect others from HIV infection. Discussions regarding the latter centred on the moral status of non-disclosure without and with safer sex practice. Throughout, participants voiced concerns over the apparently high level of disbelief and denial among the seronegative as well as personal fears of rejection.

A disclosee's need to know

Most participants at first expressed the opinion that self-disclosure was necessary with sexual partners. There were pragmatic reasons for this. Participants agreed that the last thing that they wanted was to infect others. Jon self-disclosed to his ex-partner "the day I found out because it's just – it's just my responsibility. I wouldn't put anybody's life in jeopardy for my own good." Max said, "By saying nothing, you risk their lives." Earlier, Max had said that non-disclosure was "not fair to the other person. Why put the other person through what [you] are going through?"

Maria explained:

> If your partner doesn't know. ...[Say] I'm with a man, and we've been in a relationship for years, I'm not cheating on him, he's not – we're not going out on each other: we're together. I have my tubes tied. It's not like I can get pregnant, so if I don't tell this guy he's not going to want to use a condom, and in the process he can get the virus from me.

Participants agreed that partners have a need to know about one's seropositivity because of the assumptions expressed by Maria that (a) being in a relationship renders AIDS risks null and void when neither partner is known to be HIV positive, and (b) among heterosexuals, condoms can only be legitimately used for contraception. The assumption here is that partners are monogamous and, accordingly, have known each other for some time. With casual partners, things were seen differently.

In keeping with our claims regarding social distance's role in self-disclosure decision-making, the duration and depth of the relationship in question was seen as key. Disclosure was not deemed necessary for the good of a casual relationship, and the consequences of telling new or one-time partners, who do not necessarily have one's best interests in mind, could be dire. Janie said, "You don't know the person, [or if] when they go home, are they gonna say [anything]? What are they gonna say? Where they gonna say it? To who? You don't want that [i.e. gossip]." Almost all participants promoted non-disclosure conjoined with safer sex in such situations.

As noted in Chapter 6, disclosure is generally preceded by a period of 'testing the water' to assess a disclosee's probable response, and this was the case with sexual partners just as with other social contacts. Some participants warned that one should not self-disclose until a relationship had solidified. Eddie said that the time to self-disclose was when partners decided to make commitments to each other as lovers. Joe said, "I would not disclose at first to anybody ... until that relationship had time to build so that you had something to disclose to."

As we have noted, almost every finding from one site was paralleled at the others; no exceptions were seen in the relationship data. For instance, Tony, a gay Scot, said his strategy was to disclose during the third date, which symbolized for him a certain level of commitment. At each site, participants said that such commitment is demonstrated and confirmed through acts of self-disclosure (more on this later).

Relationship ideals notwithstanding, the New Mexico data showed that disclosing in established relationships was far from straightforward. Dee described her partner's reaction to her own self-disclosure: "He's telling me to drop dead and how he was going to kill me." While such might keep many from self-disclosing, Dee felt that "I deserved whatever he would do to me." She had internalized a sense of her own danger and culpability.

After her partner "got over that level [i.e. of violent fury]," the two "went back in our tracks and asked people, 'Go get a test; it's free at Planned Parenthood.' [And they say,] 'I don't want to know'." Janie's estranged husband reacted with denial: "Up to this day he knows about it but he will not get checked. ...He says he don't have it, period."

The benefits of disclosing when the response is such may seem minimal, especially in comparison with the high costs of rejection and the very real threat of physical attack. At the same time, by 'telling', a PHA can free him- or herself from culpability to some degree: it is no longer solely the PHA's responsibility if a disclosed-to partner gets infected. Moreover, telling is implicated in ideals held for long-term relations, and a relationship itself may benefit from information sharing. We explore this later, when discussing the data from England.

Beneficent prophylaxis

Three of the 12 New Mexican participants felt certain that HIV was "given" them by particular individuals: one of these participants was raped; the other two were married to non-disclosing bisexual men.[2] All three felt great fury about their infections, which they felt they had no control over stopping. After being diagnosed, Janie self-disclosed to her estranged husband " 'cos I was angered" about his duplicity. Her self-disclosure was "an 'I want to get back at you' thing."

While Janie's rage led her to disclose, several participants said many PHAs use non-disclosure coupled with unsafe sex to express their rage. "People are going out and doing this stuff on purpose," Dee explained. "They [say,] 'Well somebody gave it to me so I'm going to give it to someone else'. That's horrible. That's murder to me."

Ron told of a seronegative friend who had said to him, "If I found out I had that, I'd be out there trying to get [i.e. infect] every [woman] I could." In telling such stories – in contrasting themselves with such "horrible" people – Dee and Ron and the others present themselves as morally upright and highly ethical. Through this strategy, PHAs may preserve self-esteem. As Ron explained, he had previously been plagued by the idea that he had not fulfilled his family's expectations; "I [thought I was] this wretched human being." The need to defend one's reputation by telling tales of even more "wretched" individuals is manifest.

Amidst the moralizing rhetoric, Rick acknowledged having had unsafe sex without self-disclosing, just like the hyperbolized HIV-positive killer does. But, he noted:

> I don't think I was necessarily having unsafe sex to hurt anybody. ...When you're doing drugs you do all kind of – your reasoning is pretty much gone. ...I reasoned it that the person that I was with probably already was infected, and I was in fact right, but it didn't ... that doesn't make it right.

Rick's move from presenting himself as a drugged man whose "reasoning [was] pretty much gone" to one having fine logic capabilities ("I reasoned it ... and I was in fact right") helped Rick and the others to accept and dismiss an act (non-disclosure) that otherwise might have been deemed a permanent stain on his character or moral record. And through his second rhetorical move – that of implicitly comparing his past self with his present, morally knowledgeable self (the self that acknowledged: "that doesn't make it right") – Rick laid a claim to being a good man capable of recognizing, admitting to, and avoiding a repeat of past indiscretions.

Joe, who is bisexual, also told of non-disclosure – to his wife. Joe rationalized his secrecy, saying he meant to inform her but had not yet identified a good time to do so. Fear of exposing homo- or bisexuality (and sometimes infidelity) to female lovers causes many closeted men to hide their seropositivity (e.g. Chiodo and Tolle 1992; Dunbar and Rehm 1992; Gard 1990). If Joe had such a fear, he did not mention it. But Max did. He held that when people learn that a man is HIV positive, they immediately ask themselves, "'Is he gay? ... Does he sleep around? Is he a big whore-dog? Does he do drugs?'" Eric summarized: "Disclosing to somebody is like sewing a scarlet letter on."

Sometimes, participants said, disclosure was unnecessary. Maria kept her sero-status secret from a number of partners, but this was conjoined with safe sex practice. She explained, "I was in and out of monogamous relationships and I'd never told them, you know? I protected, 'cos I didn't want to catch anything else, but I also knew that if I was with a man that I would protect him." In addition to sending a message regarding beneficent or altruistic safer sex practice in this statement ("I protect him"), Maria used the designation "monogamous" to confer socio-cultural legitimacy on short-term relationships. Further, she voiced her concern for her own health in addition to that of her partners. She later noted: "What people don't realize is that *we* catch things. And they're so scared of catching stuff from us. ...And they're coughing all over me and gossiping at the same time. And I'm thinking, 'Don't you know that cold can kill me'?

Participants felt that the strategy of beneficent prophylaxis (i.e. a benevolent insistence on safer sex) would negate a partner's need to know about one's sero-positivity.[3] As Joe said, "I would not disclose, but I would make sure there were no dangers [by taking] safety measures." Taking such measures would allow the PHA to reclaim higher moral ground.

Maria related an interchange she had with a male friend after meeting a man she liked:

> And I says to [my friend], "Should I tell him I'm HIV positive? I'm gonna sleep with this guy." And he's like, "I don't think you should." I says, "Well, maybe I should." He says, "Just use a condom. Just make sure you use a condom. You're not going to get in a relationship with this guy – he's married." And I thought, "OK." So I slept with him ... and I never told him.[4]

Maria started out, she claimed, with idealistic thoughts of full disclosure, but her friend showed her why this was not necessary. Similarly, Dee said, "[People] tell me, 'Girl, if I was you I wouldn't tell!'"

Most participants describing sex with casual partners spoke of non-disclosure coupled with safer sex. Janie proclaimed, "I don't say, but I do take precautions"; Rick declared, "I don't tell, but [I do] protect." However, most participants reported that they were not always so punctilious in actuality. And some lamented that, even when they were, their partners' behaviour did not change.

Disbelief and denial among the seronegative

Many participants said that despite high levels of AIDS awareness among the lay-public (and high knowledge levels do exist, even among the disenfranchised; e.g. Harrison *et al.* 1991; Jemmott and Jemmott 1991) partners often chose to forgo protection. Participants sometimes understood this as stemming from foolish human nature: Ron argued, "Human beings are human beings and they're still going to do the same stupid shit that got us into this shit anyway." But most participants felt that because AIDS knowledge is high (or perceived to be so) a partner's refusal to use condoms must stem from informed personal choice:

Maria: The majority of people know about AIDS...

Joe: But haven't you run into a situation where they may know but they may not care?

Maria: Yeah, I have.

Joe: I mean, there's that point. I mean, people are educated to some degree about HIV and AIDS ... and although they may know, they'll take the risk anyway.

Maria: That's true, that's very true.

Joe: So I mean if at that point in time – It just depends, I have said that sometimes I do [tell] and sometimes I don't. When I have [told and] the other person knows full well and they choose not take any safety measures, that decision is totally up to them. That's their decision.

Likewise, Janie said, "If a person's willing to have sex and just do it ... OK" [i.e. that's their decision]. But Eric said that you "can't assume somebody else's knowledge [and so you have] to accept responsibility" [i.e. insist on protection].[5]

Ron noted, "It's very difficult to negotiate for safe sex." Janie agreed: "It's not easy, because my partner – well my partner doesn't like using condoms, and I get afraid because I know the importance of it, and yet he doesn't, so he doesn't seem to see." Later, Janie explained,

> They don't like using condoms, and right off the bat they say, "Well I don't have AIDS." That's the first thing: "I don't have AIDS." And I go, "I didn't say you did," and then they say, "I had myself checked two months ago" [which shows that they really do not understand the disease] but you don't want to go into detail with them, because by that time they wonder, "Well why are you so up to date on that stuff?"

Maria pointed out, "Most men do not accept women being HIV positive. It's a difficult thing for them, I guess because it's [perceived as] a gay [male] disease." (Chapter 11 examines the different experiences of men and women, gays and straights, and hemophiliacs and IDUs; here, our focus is partner disbelief in general.)

According to participants, besides failing to internalize the safer sex message and so denying their own risks for AIDS, people also harbour disbelief when explicitly disclosed to. Maria, diagnosed in the mid-eighties, said:

> [My ex-partner], through the whole entire time, did not believe me; for years, never believed me. "Ah, you're full of it." He'd always tell me that. He didn't believe me and we never protected each other and I kept always telling him. ...He didn't believe me until the guy who takes the blood – what are they called? He came in to draw my blood and he put two pairs of gloves on and [my ex] says, "Why you wearing all those gloves?" " 'Cos she's HIV positive." [My partner's] eyes got this big around! I mean, he was sitting in his chair and he was like [sits straight up] "What?!" And just jumped out of his chair, and I looked at him, and I said, "What? Do you think I've been lying to you for six years? I've been telling you for years."

To feel normal again

When asked if most PHAs self-disclosed to sexual partners, Max, who was not sexually active at the time of his participation, told us, "Most people pretend they don't have it ... not on purpose, but to feel normal again. They want to stay with a healthy point of view rather than to be thinking about [AIDS] all the time. " Max said that PHAs "go back to being normal" when "they pretend it's not there". Beyond self-conscious 'pretending', he said, many think that if they "take another blood test it won't be there; it was a mistake or misunderstanding" (more of which later).

Max spoke of his own "human" desire for a "feeling of being not alone; feeling wanted." Non-disclosure appeared to Max as a way to gratify those desires, while in disclosing "you take the chance of them leaving. [But] you need the affection of somebody else other than family or friends. You are lonely, and scared you're gonna die."

Acceptance and rejection

"Acceptance and rejection. That's the two main issues," declared Maria. Despite widespread fear of the latter, Meg said, "There's people that I know who have told their partners and they're still in relationships." On telling her own partner, Meg said, "I was scared to, because I didn't know if he was going to leave me or if he was just gonna like stay with me for a little while and then leave or just leave me right then and there." He stayed. So did Jon's partner, who, Jon said, "was very supportive of me. We stayed together for quite a while."

Maria encountered rejection from neither her current primary partner nor from her past one:

> You know, even after my [then-boyfriend] found out – I mean for sure knew that I was HIV positive, it still never mattered to him. This guy was so in love with me. His thing was, "If you're going to die, we'll die together." I thought, "That's the ultimate." Yeah. That's kinda like the Romeo and Juliet thing, you know. ...[He stood by me], knowing still I was HIV positive.

Maria's reference to "the Romeo and Juliet thing" indexes a cultural model of love that many participants aspired to, and fits with research regarding the significance of unsafe sex as symbolic of love and devotion (Sobo 1993a, 1995b). Her initial remarks bespeak a fear that HIV infection entails an end to all intimacy if revealed. But her story demonstrates that although "it can cost us for telling someone," self-disclosure success does happen.

Only two of the 12 participants, Dee and Joe, reported immediate rejection from a primary partner. In Joe's case, it was his wife, who learned of his condition from an outside source. Her rejection lessened over time and patterns of interaction were re-established as acceptance grew. The same was true for Dee. But in other cases, hurts did not mend. And, as Joe pointed out, rejection wasn't always immediate: "When I chose to disclose to [a steady lover, he] would at first say it was OK, yet the more that [we were] in the relationship ... there were other issues that came out, [from] down below." Joe's partner was slowly shutting down on him emotionally; he "was having a hard time. ...He felt 'I cannot love you because you are HIV positive; I cannot feel more than that'. And that's restricting."

Joe felt that self-disclosure often ignites a long process of emotional work in partners. His wife and he talk, Joe said, but only "surface talk, surface talk. ...They're going through their own set of issues. ...They may have issues that they haven't totally [discovered] because it's a process, it's a learning process."

Joe also said, "They will want to isolate you, they want you all to themselves. But they want to isolate you [also because] they don't want anybody else to know that you're HIV positive." Maria added, "They're embarrassed of the idea of a lover being HIV."

Six of the 12 participants were partnered at the time of the study. Janie, who felt encouraged by the success stories she heard in the focus group discussion, had just begun dating a man and had not yet disclosed to him. "I'm afraid that if he'd know he might not want to be with me or spend time with me," she said, explaining:

> I don't have anybody to really be a mate, a companion; I don't have that. So when I think about it, it hurts. You just think that you don't have nothing to live for. ...You say to yourself, "Are you ever going to be involved with anybody? Is anybody going to accept you? Are they going to want you once they find out? Are they going to have a life with you?"

Janie's words, like those reported earlier for Max, were a plea for normalcy. When describing her experience of disclosing to a new partner – the person she is still with – Maria said,

> We dated for about two weeks and we were kinda getting close. It was really hard for me. "No, I'm not going to tell yet; yeah I'll tell; no I'm not going to tell." And I thought, like, "I can't give it to him." And I went back and forth with it, and I just kinda started eating up inside about it. And then finally I just said "Hey, I'm HIV positive; how do you feel about this?" So he got out of the truck and went to the bathroom in the gas station and came back and he was just looking at me, like, "What?" "Well, I just told you something." "Oh, I love you, it's OK." I was like, "*What?*" I expected rejection. [Meg interjects: So did I.] I really expected to be rejected, like, "Oh my God how can you do this?" Or, "Ooh I don't want to be a part of *that*."

The fear of rejection is paramount, and the struggle to decide to disclose ("Yeah I'll tell; no I'm not going to tell") is clear.

Rejection can come from within as well as from without. Eric's hypothetical advice to seronegative partners of PHAs, "Get out while you can," bespeaks such self-rejection. Participants in both focus groups raised the question of partnering with other PHAs, who might be more sympathetic and with whom one might be able to be more candid.

For example, Rick said, "I prefer – I feel better about it [i.e. partnering with PHAs]. It's probably not better for you or anything [but] I feel more comfortable with it. I feel it gets that stuff out of the way. It is an issue still, but it's not like a big disclosure."

In the other group, the question was raised by Joe and taken up by Maria, who said:

> I don't think I can have a relationship with someone that's positive, actually I couldn't. [It would be a] turn off. To me, I'm healthy; to me, I'm kinda normal. ...And if I got into a relationship with someone else that was HIV positive my whole world would be HIV positive, because I got to deal with someone else that was HIV positive and I would have to deal with their issues about being HIV positive and I couldn't do that. ...[Plus,] I would be scared of catching something [all laugh]!

Partnering with another PHA would undermine Maria's ability to feel "kinda normal".

North-East England: more of the same?

The issues raised by New Mexican participants also emerged in the two British studies. Indeed, although there was some difference in emphasis, perhaps largely due to differences in the approach taken by each study, the similarity of the issues raised and the moral positions voiced by participants in all three samples was remarkable. In presenting the English data, then, we focus on the ways in which relationship ideals affect self-disclosure decisions and expectations.

The relationship ideal in England

All eight English participants, straight and gay, subscribed to a mainstream relationship ideal of caring commitment, honesty and trust. As Chuck proclaimed, "If there's no trust there's no point in having a relationship." Trust demanded disclosing serostatus information about oneself, and trust meant feeling safe in that disclosure. By definition, having an intimate primary relationship meant being able – and willing – to share serostatus information. Whether legal spouses or, as was more commonly the case, long-term boy- or girlfriends, or newer but committed partners slated for a long-term partner role, primary partners had a need to know based on the level of emotional intimacy that had been reached with them. Jamie explained:

You reach a point in a relationship where you have built up sufficient trust in each other and you have some sort of – you have worked some relationship out and it is fairly stable. ...And I think [by not sharing] you would end up being underhand and deceitful and whatever that's about that's not a good thing whether it would be HIV or anything else in a relationship.

Put more simply, "If you love somebody and you're in a relationship you share everything with them." Self-disclosure sometimes even served as a 'performative', itself establishing a relationship as a relatively stable entity.[6] The intimacy that conjugality in our culture entails serves not only to help create and reinforce the relationship but also to help maintain and reinforce the self, providing a point of coherence for it. As Cancian notes in relation to love, "A stable self is a social product that develops out of enduring relationships, and shared beliefs and values" (Cancian 1987: 149). In any case, up until a person felt sure that a relationship had staying power, self-disclosure was perceived as quite a gamble. Frank's answer to our question regarding whether he had a responsibility to disclose demonstrates the complex nature of the decision: "Yeah, well yeah, well no, well yeah and no, I feel, you see how can I put it?"

Frank later said "If I told him and it might only last two or three months and we finish then everybody knows about me." Jamie, who had similar fears, weighed them against his relationship ideals when he described his feelings for a man who had recently won his heart but to whom he had yet to disclose:

He said em "If you love somebody you stick by them don't you?" But I don't know. ...If he's committed like he says he is and if he says the trust and all the things he's said, he sticks by – well then everything hopefully should work out and I'll be able to sit back once in life and go [sighs] "thank God for that," and just get on with your life and be happy and all the rest of it, have a little picket fence and all.

All participants valued love relationships, and Jamie's reference to a "picket fence" indexed his at least partial adherence to a mainstream model of conjugality. While many gay men may adhere to this model, such adherence may be more likely in more rural, less cosmopolitan regions, where attitudes may be more old-fashioned and partnering options more limited.

Beneficent prophylaxis and responsibility for one's own health

Disclosure decisions were more straightforward when love and expectations for truthfulness and real emotional intimacy did not enter the equation. As for the New Mexicans, self-disclosure for North-East England participants was not mandatory or even recommended in casual relationships. It was assumed that casual partners would have high levels of AIDS knowledge and expected that they would take responsibility for their own health due to the known risks of having unsafe sex on one-night stands.

Timothy said that people he meets for such "must somehow be aware because they are going out, they are actively looking for sex therefore sex is an issue for them and therefore HIV must be an issue for them". That is, they should know better than to have unprotected sex with strangers. And Frank said,

> "At the end of the day [a sexual partner] should be considering himself because he's responsible for his own well being and if he isn't prepared to do that, well then, if he did catch anything well then unfortunately that's down to him. He can't blame anybody else."

While some have suggested that the English might not be as receptive as US citizens to the rhetoric of others' personal responsibility for themselves,[7] such rhetoric did come up quite often in participants' discourse.

At the same time, participants did feel a need to recommend prophylaxis: Malcolm said, "As long as I take the initiative in safer sex em, because I have the knowledge of what I'm carrying then I'm all right morally in my books." Likewise, Bob said, "Since I knew that I was HIV, now before you start making love I say 'Well I will put one on' but if she says 'No' that's it; at least you have told her before you started."

Not all rhetoric about trying to impose safer sex centred on protecting partners; Chuck said, "Really I should make him put a condom on to protect myself from him, he could have the virus and I could have two strains then." Perhaps due to the influences of available written material or local counselling jargon, concern for one's own health in England centred on infection with another 'strain' of HIV while New Mexicans' concerns were voiced more in terms of the death-dealing capacity of the 'common cold'. The Scots voiced concern about both.

Condoms: distasteful and abnormal

Despite public knowledge, all participants reported encountering resistance to suggestions regarding safer sex. For one thing, not everyone enjoys using condoms. People reported both personal distaste for them, the distaste of others, and a desire to avoid the distressing reminder of one's lack of so-called normalcy that condom use can entail.

Regarding female condoms, Kevin said "They are crap, horrible things, bin [trash can] liners." Matthew talked about what he and his companions thought of male condoms: "We don't like using them. None of us can use them and come so we don't use them at all."

Jamie suggested, "I don't think it would interfere with the mechanics. I think it is more to do with the emotional trust, that side of things, rather than the actual [sex]." Chuck explained:

> If you don't wear a condom then you, you, it, you think to yourself like you're not HIV and you're no different to anybody else so I think, I can understand people that do have sex with people that don't wear condoms because it's – it removes that black cloud that you're carrying around with you ... it's as though you're normal, do you know what I mean? You've got nothing to hide and nothing to worry about, the next day I mean the guilt trip's so bad but er I can understand people that don't have safer sex with other people.

Chuck positions himself as one who knows right from wrong, even as he shows sympathy for the plight of those who stray, casting the desire for unsafe sex as very human. Although he does not directly claim to have had unsafe sex himself, he certainly implies that he has done so. Indeed, feeling normal (i.e. not seropositive) is so important to him that, he said, if someone other than his primary partner asked him to put a condom on, "I'd probably say 'Why?' That's nasty isn't it?"

Risk denial and disbelief

In England as in New Mexico, participants thought partners often refused condoms because they failed to see their own risks for HIV infection. Most of the participants had no sympathy for this because, at least in relation to strangers, and at least in certain contexts, they subscribed to media messages casting those who get infected due to a lack of prophylaxis as stupid. Once, when responding to a PHA who

155

claimed not to have known about safer sex, Frank said, "'Well that's rubbish.' I said, 'There was loads of stuff out that was on em the television, posters, all this 'Don't die of ignorance'. I said, 'You can't say that you didn't know,' I said, 'because it [information] was there'."

But, perhaps due not to ignorance but to partner denial, stemming from self-esteem needs and cognitive biases (Sobo 1995b; Weinstein 1989), many participants reported that partners frequently refused protection. Matthew had a way to offset this: "[What] I have done before when someone asked me not to use one. ...I just said 'Yeah all right I won't bother then' but then put a condom on while he was bent over and fucked him and he didn't really know."

Even partners aware of the participants' serostatus sometimes refused to take protective measures. Kevin told his girlfriend when he was diagnosed; "She knows it but she just says that, 'You haven't got it, you have not got it,' and denies it." Kevin generally insisted on condoms, but she often begged him to forgo them.

> We went to bed and were cuddling and having a bit of a smooch and everything and I went to the drawer and got a condom out. She said, "No don't use one." I said "Eh?" She said, "Don't use one, just this once." I said "Don't be daft." She said, "It is alright." I said, "It is not alright."

Kevin spontaneously suggested that "she was maybe doing it so I would feel as if I could still do it without a condom if you know what I mean ... out of love."

Findings from the Scottish data are relevant here. One-half of the 62 Scottish participants who were asked were in primary relationships; 23 with people who had not to their partner's knowledge tested HIV positive and eight with other PHAs. The decision to have unsafe sex among serodiscordant couples was reportedly made by the HIV-negative partner and in many cases against the wishes of the positive partner. However, all but two of the participants with seropositive partners preferred unprotected sex, at least on some occasions. They felt that cross-infection was a small risk compared to the benefits of unrestricted sexual behaviour.

It is clear from all three research sites that, with primary partners, decisions about the relationship *per se* often were given higher priority than the risk of HIV transmission. Some participants reported that their partners encouraged them to have penetrative sex without condoms in order to make them feel more comfortable with and committed to the relationship. Others mentioned that their partners wanted children or felt that HIV was a joint problem.

Relationship ideals foster AIDS-risk denial among the uninfected

In support of, and because of, trust and love, and in keeping with mainstream under-standings regarding conjugal partnering, unsafe sexual activity in the context of a primary relationship was expected. The assumption that one should not have to protect oneself from one's primary partner, pervasive among US women (Kinsey 1994; Sobo 1993a, 1995b), was common among the Englishmen. It affected not only partner responses but participants' own risk-related sexual decisions, both before and after testing positive.

Take, for example, Chuck's declaration: "I didn't used to have safer sex 'cos I was in a relationship, wasn't I." When his doctor asked him to consider an HIV test, he replied, "Don't be so stupid ... I can't possibly have HIV. ...It was just me and [my partner, monogamously] all the time." Jamie also felt, pre-diagnosis, that his relationship with his primary partner was safe: "He said he'd only been with, he'd been with Rob for 20-odd years and he'd never ever been with anybody else." Further:

> He was like really clued up on things ... and so I figured well you know, he's so observant and so careful. ...I suppose in a way he had like conned me in not to wear condoms if you see what I mean. "Oh there's no need for you to do that, there's no need." ...I think I was more besotted with him, so I was like "Oh anything he says you know is 100 per cent" so if he told me to stick my head in a fire I probably would have done it.

In hindsight, Jamie cast himself as the quintessential fool for love.

Supporting one's relationship: variations on the theme

Jamie, Chuck, and some other North-Easterners did expect partners to engage in sex outside of a primary relationship but they also expected them to be "careful" when doing so. Timothy explained that outside sex, and threesomes, are "reasonably common 'cos it is one way of people to keep their relationships fresh". This model justifies outside sex as something beneficial and structurally functional (provided that care is taken to protect the health of one's primary partner, whether through actual risk reduction (e.g. safer sex) or perceived risk reduction (e.g. through 'wise' partner choice; see Sobo 1993a, 1995b). Indeed, it is not only acceptable, it is essential, for the good of the relationship.[8]

157

Relationship expectations and denial of risk status

We did not explicitly query mode of infection and we certainly did not require explanations. Yet all of the men at one point or another told us that they believed their risks for infection to be low prior to testing positive; many saw their infections as exceptions. They offered what we call 'alternate explanations' for infection. These seemed to be tied to their relationship expectations and those they held for primary partners, and in some cases they were directly linked to the recasting of risky actions as being 'for the benefit of the relationship'. Self-expectations for morality tied to sexual and relationship ideals also came into play.

In a typical alternate explanation, Frank declared:

> I'm not trying to get out of it but I didn't, quite honestly I didn't feel that I had done anything what had put me at risk but obviously it had, but I hadn't done anything sexually through the main lines like either having anal intercourse or, or injecting drugs, I've never done any of that.

In an explanation that was more unique but similarly useful in terms of moral posturing, Malcolm said, "I don't know if I contracted it via sexual contact; it would have been fairly difficult 'cos I've always followed safer sex practice."[9] Malcolm then conjectured that he was infected "because I worked as a volunteer in an HIV unit", constructing himself as a good person and innocent victim to boot. He sought to establish a route of infection whereby, as he said, "it wasn't my fault."

Each of the men interviewed felt that he'd been careful. Each (perhaps barring Matthew, for reasons explained below) was surprised to be infected with HIV. This surprise was probably genuine; optimistically biased appraisal of one's risk for a preventable disease seems to be common among people of all walks of life (Weinstein 1987). Because of a fairly simple cognitive bias related especially to the perception that HIV infection is preventable if one lives up to cultural expectations regarding conjugal relations (*cf.* Sobo 1995b: 33–37), others are seen as less careful than oneself. For example, Malcolm noted that many people can be quite defensive regarding their risks for HIV:

> They don't want to confront the possibility that their behaviour ... they sort of say "I wasn't that promiscuous really" sort of the minute the HIV question comes up they are worried but they straight away sort of, a double blindness ... like "I wasn't that bad."

By maintaining claims to irregular modes of infection in the form of alternate explanations, PHAs present themselves as innocent, or good – as still being worthy of esteem and status or at least the respect of their fellow human beings.

Another way to maintain moral personhood is to write one's infection off to chance in the scientific sense of the term. Two of the eight participants did just that. It remains to be seen what predisposes people to decouple morality from the infection equation. It may be that homosexual men who are active members of cosmopolitan-style gay communities are more likely to see infection as something beyond one's control or as having little to do with goodness or badness *per se*. As one such Englishman said, "The gay community just passes it off as, 'Well that's it, anyone could get it at any time, it is just a risk that's there and if you got it then that's it'." Disinterest in one's mode of infection also may reflect a desire to spend only a minimum of time thinking about one's status as a PHA.

A third tactic regarding morality and mode of infection, and the tactic we are most interested in in the context of this chapter, is to cast one's seroconversion as symbolic of one's commitment to one's partner. Unsafe sex can occur among discordant couples when the seronegative partner seeks to support the seropositive one in a way that is in keeping with relationship ideals. That is, one of the things that seronegative partners can do for love is to offer seropositive partners unsafe sex (as in the previously mentioned "Romeo and Juliet thing").

Recalling his seronegative days, Matthew said, "I remember nagging at [my partner] sort of like saying, 'I don't want to use them I want to give you something that other people won't give you. I am going out with you and I love you so much'." Matthew explained, albeit with some regret, "I wanted HIV because I wanted to share what he was feeling. ...I don't want to be here when he is not." Matthew eventually seroconverted. He and his partner were planning a wedding when he last spoke with his interviewer.

Many gay men may look forward to a version of marriage or, as Jamie earlier described it, "a little picket fence and all". But little has been written about how mainstream (heterosexual) relationship ideals affect gay men's negotiation of sexual risks. It may be that seropositive gay men are more apt to be swayed by mainstream ideals because of their changed circumstances. More research in this area is called for if we are to chart the varied landscapes of risk that PHAs face.

Acceptance and rejection after self-disclosure

Once disclosed to, partners often needed time to digest the news. Malcolm explained that the "confrontational approach in disclosure is not necessarily the best, em, exposure because people don't have time to think about what their reaction's going to be. ...They don't have time to cool off, they don't have time to em analyse or, or consider their standpoint." This and the popularity of the testing-the-waters strategy notwithstanding, several participants reported unplanned, explosive self-disclosures. Generally, these followed a stressful period of rumination capped with a triggering event.

For example, Chuck disclosed when his primary partner Jay accused him of infidelity. He had intended to tell Jay of his diagnosis, but the relationship was new, and he hadn't yet confirmed for himself, through conversational fishing, that his new partner's reaction would be favourable or, indeed, that this partnership was good for the long term. At the time, he said,

> I was still seeing this other lad [Ben]. ...There had been rumours going round that I was seeing [Jay] and all that and I said, "No we're just friends" and all that and [Ben] said, "Don't forget what you are," and it was like blackmailing us. ...I ended up having sex with [Ben] ... and really all I did it for was to try and stop him from telling [Jay] before I wanted to tell him first.

Jay soon found out about Chuck's liaison with Ben through the grapevine, Chuck said:

> so I got myself absolutely mortal drunk. ...We were driving home and he says, "What did you have sex with him for?" I said "Oh Jay" I says "You don't understand ... to stop, he's blackmailing us." He says, "What for?" I say, "I'm HIV," just like that. Well, he nearly crashed the car ... I was just crying my eyeballs out, and I got home, got to his house and he just ... he was just like absolutely fabulous with – I went to bed and I cried myself to sleep and em the next morning and he was just looking at us, he was sat up, he said, "Do you know I haven't slept at all, I've been awake all night long," he says ... "just looking at you." I says, "Oh." He says em, he says "I can't get over it." I says, "You can't get over it?" I say, "You don't realize what I've gone through." ...I said, "I was so frightened of him telling you." ..."I've fallen in love with you," he says; "It makes no difference to me now that you're like that."

As in most successful disclosures to primary partners, love underwrote Jay's acceptance of Chuck's condition. Chuck's success was not seamless: safer sex still posed a problem. But Chuck's success was no less real for this. His partner's commitment was deep; he supported Chuck emotionally, and maintained a sense of humour and an understanding outlook. Seven of the eight English participants experienced what we call 'authentic successes'.[10]

Some success was, in contrast, 'inauthentic success'; beneath a superficial facade of acceptance, rejection festered. Delayed or tacit rejection responses like those reported earlier for some of the New Mexican participants also were reported in England. For example, Timothy had a partner with whom, he said:

> I could sense and see physical movements back from him. Tiny, tiny physical movements and he didn't want to kiss me at certain points or you could feel that he was kind of like – I am very sensitive to body movements. ...He wouldn't touch. ...He didn't want me to use a razor because of the fear of me micro-cutting myself, nicks and stuff like that. Blood; blood the poison. So I went with it and he bought me an electric razor and I hated it. Each and every day I shaved with this fucking thing it kept on acting as a reminder and it kept on saying to me you have got to change your whole life all the time.

When Timothy was advised, "Go back to wet shaving, get rid of [that] boyfriend because there are plenty of fish in the sea," he said that "My perspective of it were, there were certainly not any fish in the sea at all." He felt at the time "that I have really no right to choose quality any longer; I had to put up with what ever came my way, simply because anybody who could put up with me being positive was good enough." Timothy's identification with the negative connotations of AIDS led to feelings of insufficiency and a low tolerance for the risk of relationship loss.

Delayed and tacit rejection was also reported by the Scottish participants. Heather, for example, told her new partner about her drug use shortly after meeting him, and revealed her HIV status a week later:

> Well when the relationship first started I told him about myself and things and I thought he was really understandable, but then after a month or so he changed, he just – it was like he was still coming to see me and things but he started to like – oh he just stopped like, we stopped having sex. He used to make excuses, and then eventually it got to the stage where he was even scared to kiss me. It was a right let down, you know. It took me months to get over it. ...It'll take me a long time to trust a man again.

161

In both British studies participants remarked on the power imbalances that tended to emerge among discordant couples, along with over-dependency or over-commitment on the part of one partner. A young Scot, Michael, who had recently come through a harrowing decoupling told us:

> If someone decides knowing I am HIV positive to sleep with me I feel they are making a major commitment that normally you would not do if you were sleeping with somebody. They are taking extra commitment. It is easier for me because there is no risk for me. ...That is why [Jane] and I lasted so long in the end. ...There was a lot of emotional blackmail which was HIV-related and which maintained the relationship for a year longer than it would normally have gone on. It made it a lot more extreme and a lot more intense, and a lot more problematic. Just crazy basically, it got to crazy levels which would never have happened if it had not been for HIV.

Disequilibrium perpetuated relationships that might otherwise have ended. It also fostered guilt. Participants expressed guilt about being ill or being dependent on their partners and felt worried about their potential for infecting them. In North-East England, Malcolm had a partner with whom "if anything did sort of reach boundary level of un-safe he would put me onto a tremendous guilt trip after to deliberately manipulate that and sort of use it to, to sort of coerce me into, into giving him gifts and things." Although emotional blackmail is not uncommon in relationships in general, when AIDS enters the equation interactions can be more damaging than usual, due to the impact they have on the HIV-related identity constructions of the PHA.

The following example, provided by English participant Chuck, is perhaps a bit extreme but it shares many elements with more typical unbalanced relationship stories:

> I once told a lad who I was in a relationship a year and a half and he stuck with us. ...The only reason I think he stayed with us was because er he was hoping I was going to be dying shortly and leaving him everything ... and he had me going to a solicitor's [US: lawyer's] with him to do, change all my will over to him. ...He made us em make a living will as well where he had complete control. A year later ... I told him I was selling up and ... he went crazy on us. ...[I] completely regret telling him 'cos I mean he even phoned up the biggest gossip woman in the village and told her. ...It was devastating.

Horrible people

While partners can be awful, so too can PHAs. Participants themselves mostly tried to protect their partners from infection, but all had heard of others who would not. Like the New Mexicans, the English participants wrote such PHAs off as evil or deranged: "That is not a typical person it is just a psycho." At the same time, they contrasted themselves with these people and demonstrated that they were good, caring, upright citizens.

Frank told his interviewer, a fellow Brit:

> [I] read something today where this woman, she's gonna actually be on the television. ...[She's] contracted AIDS and she's come out with a thing now saying that she will kill or infect a thousand men before she dies. ...They're calling her the 'angel of death'. ...I don't know where she's from, but they've got this picture and they're saying beware of this woman, yeah. Got to be an American. ...I feel sorry for her in a way because I think it's anger again: she's so angry ... but then again, I don't know. If people catch her I think she should be put down [to death] or something like that.

Frank shows that he is sensitive and caring, claiming empathy for the woman, but he also demonstrates a willingness to take drastic actions (capital punishment) to protect his fellow citizens from the threat she poses.

At the time the Scottish interviews were being conducted, the papers ran a head-lining story about a young man with haemophilia who had knowingly infected four women. His actions were roundly condemned by all the study participants with haemophilia. Opinions of him ranged from describing him as "a bit of a dot [idiot]" to "he deserves shooting." All participants were keen to distance the man and his actions from themselves.

Back in England, taking the role of the benevolent father figure, Kevin implicitly compared himself with a PHA he knew personally who was not just vindictive, but a pederast to boot:

> I know a bloke who got found HIV positive and he used to work in a club where I used to drink and he used to prey on the young kids, having sex with them unprotected. ...He thought he has got it so why shouldn't they. ...He went out and did it on purpose ... [I told him] If he does it again I will chop it off. I told the kids to get themselves checked. "Go to the hospital and get yourself checked son."

163

By his words and deeds, Kevin helped to protect the next generation from those evil PHAs who would give others a bad name by striving to spread their disease. He demonstrated that while he, too, was infected with HIV he was still a good and upright citizen.

Changing landscapes of risks reported in Scotland

Interviews in Scotland did not include direct questions on horror stories or cultural stereotypes, and they did not focus on self-disclosure to sexual partners *per se*. However, as seen above, the participants did have relevant stories to tell. They were interviewed annually over a three-year period; their stories thus provide a longitudinal perspective in addition to retrospective recall or contemporary, cross-sectional data, and thus shed further light on the shifting landscapes of risk within which sexual relationships progressed over time. Further, data from the seronegative sample provides comparison figures, helping us to understand the objective nature of certain of the PHAs' proclaimed social risks.[11]

Ineligibility

Relationship ideals differ from culture to culture but across all sites participants endorsed the establishment and maintenance of primary relationships through the trusting sharing of personal information. Members of the Scottish sample were no exception. Notwithstanding, 50 per cent of the seropositive Scottish participants were not in relationships during the first interview and this proportion remained about the same in subsequent interviews, although it was not always the same individuals at each interview who were partnered. In comparison, 50 per cent of the seronegative participants were also unpartnered.

The great majority of the partnerless, whether PHAs or members of the seronegative sample, expressed a desire to have a regular committed partnership and felt singlehood was a source of loneliness, social isolation and discontent. However, the PHAs felt ineligible as long-term partners because of the limits on their life span. They felt they could not plan a future or have a family, as this would risk transmitting the virus to partners and future children. Mitch explained, "You could have safe sex but at the end of the day it is whether you can carry on and settle down and get married and have children. That is what you want in life."

The psychological cost associated with feelings of ineligibility was extremely high. Not only did these participants feel debarred from having fulfilling committed sexual relationships, they were also denied a much-desired expected future life trajectory.

Shifting perceptions of eligibility

Seven of the 18 participants who had initially believed themselves 'ineligible' had formed long-term relationships by subsequent interviews one or two years later. One began an intense and very committed relationship with someone with another chronic illness; two formed relationships with people who worked in the HIV field; another met an HIV-positive partner; three negotiated relationships in which sex was exclusively non-penetrative.

Five participants experienced other changes in relationship status and feelings of eligibility. Janice stopped having sex with her husband after a condom burst; he later left her. Carl experienced the death of his partner and subsequently felt ineligible to enter a new partnership. Three who had been keen to find a partner at the first interview felt at later interviews that their deterioration in health made them ineligible and beside they were no longer interested.

These stories illustrate the association between perceived eligibility and landscape of risk. Landscape changes – such as when a condom bursts, a lover dies, health deteriorates, someone who knows one's serostatus says they want to have a relationship, one realizes that there is sex without penetration – these changes trigger a reassessment of one's eligibility. In this manner, a shifting risk landscape may lead to redefinitions of, and changes in, aspects of one's identity.

Intimate disclosures and social risk

The small size and regional specificity of our samples notwithstanding, we suggest that the attitudes and experiences that we have described are not especially unique. While the stories provided by members of each sample are influenced to some degree by local conditions and by each person's life history, they differ very little overall. Certain aspects of the experience of PHAs, at least in economically developed nations, seem very universal indeed.

Duration and depth of relationship

Regardless of gender, age, sexual orientation, class, or nationality, most participants shared a model for primary sexual relationships as entailing and being maintained through trust and sharing. Such relationships generally were striven for. Participants advocated self-disclosure to sexual partners on a need-to-know basis, and for most this hinged on the duration and depth of the relationship in question. While primary partners definitely had a need to know, casual partners had not earned that need.

Participants felt that beneficent prophylaxis removed any budding need to know for casual partners or when the cost of self-disclosing was likely to outweigh any benefit. The fact that many untested or seronegative individuals deny their own AIDS risks (see Kinsey 1994; Sobo 1993a, 1994, 1995b), and that partners often request unsafe sex as part of a relationship building and maintenance strategy, sometimes made this a difficult scheme to implement.

Participants primarily feared rejection, relationship loss, loss of control over serostatus information, and the loss of a sense of normalcy via disclosure. The recommended method for evaluating the likelihood of such problems involved making indirect allusions to stigmatized lifestyles or conditions and then evaluating reactions. While authentic successes in which self-disclosure met acceptance were common, inauthentic successes, in which rejection was delayed, hidden or tacit, did occur. Participants noted that even those who overtly accept their disclosures can harbour surreptitious fears. Moreover, they can revoke or threaten to revoke acceptance at later points in time, sometimes obliquely, as by using other issues as ruses for partial or complete rejection of the discloser. They can make acceptance conditional, using serostatus information in power and dependency games, often limiting the PHA's ability to form other social and sexual relationships, sometimes extending a relationship beyond its natural lifespan.

People can and do keep their seropositivity a secret from some sexual partners. However, the idea that many people do so in order to infect others would appear to reflect public paranoia and the media sensationalism that feeds it rather than factual reality (see also Chapter 2). Most who did not 'tell' in the first instance, but meant to tell later were unable to tell because of fears for their own well being, or took active steps to prevent HIV transmission to partners.

Rumours of angry PHAs who conceal their seropositivity with the malicious intent of spreading HIV circulate in Britain and the USA, and although PHAs may point to media sensationalism, they do not deny that some PHAs do resort to such practices. And comparing oneself to such vindictive people helps demonstrate and even create one's own moral superiority over other PHAs and one's moral equality with one's interlocutor or members of the community to which one would like to belong.

Balancing risks

Research to date has shown that a number of people from all transmission groups at least occasionally practise unsafe sex and risk transmitting the virus to seronegative partners (Dublin *et al*. 1992; Green 1994a; 1995b; Hankins *et al*. 1993; Johnstone *et al*. 1990; Weatherburn 1993; White *et al*. 1993). However, knowingly exposing others to the virus most often occurs within the context of a loving committed relationship in which sexual partners are fully aware of the risk or a casual relationship in which sexual partners are seen as educated adults, free to choose non-protection if they wish.

It has been suggested that many people disregard the risk of HIV in sexual relationships because loving or even simply knowing someone can lead people to assume that they are 'clean' and safe (e.g. Weatherburn *et al*. 1991; Ingham *et al*. 1991; Sobo 1995b). The value people place on personal relationships and related feelings of solidarity or affection and trust between partners often overrides concern with HIV infection. Maintenance of personal relationships may transcend concern with HIV transmission as a risk, and it may be that this is even more important for PHAs than for seronegative or untested individuals, due to their generally more precarious sense of hold on physical and social life.

Fear of rejection and relationship loss often underlies a PHA's silence regarding his or her serostatus. But our research shows that such negative outcomes are far from routine. Other research findings also suggest that PHAs can, we think due to internalization of a negative or dangerous PHA identity or identity component, overestimate the likelihood of rejection. Findings from a Los Angeles study carried out with 684 ethnically diverse men indicated that self-disclosers received more favourable reactions than they expected, and that reactions were generally supportive (Mansergh *et al*. 1995). A study involving 65 ethnically diverse women also revealed generally positive outcomes (Simoni *et al*. 1995). And a project comparing experiences of seropositive men with those of seronegatives found that 82 per cent of seropositive men who self-disclosed to primary partners reported six months later that their relationships remained "as strong as ever". Only 70 per cent of seronegative men who self-disclosed their test results reported the same (Schnell *et al*. 1992).

The questionable nature of concern over rejection notwithstanding, avoidance of rejection is not the only motivation for sexual risk taking. Risks to sexual health are also overridden by the desire to conceive; safer sex is incompatible with the reproductive affirmation of life. And sometimes, what others might call 'high-risk' behaviour is actually a more attractive, less risky option than taking preventive measures. Sobo (1993a, 1995b) has shown that unsafe sex implies closeness, trust, honesty and commitment and signals successful participation in an ideal relationship. Very similar patterns of thought underlie some of the unsafe sex reported by the

PHAs in our Scottish, English, and New Mexican samples, whether they have hetero-sexual or homosexual relations. And the relationship ideals that drive unsafe sex also can drive self-disclosure: under certain conditions of commitment, sharing serostatus information actually helps to create or maintain a relationship's quality and stability.

It is clear that HIV-risk behaviour can only be understood within context, using a holistic framework. In participants' eyes, each individual has to balance the risk of transmitting HIV or picking up sickness against social and psychological risks, including risks for relationships and self-esteem, that may accompany safer sex or full disclosure of one's serostatus. The possibility of infecting a partner or being subject to public disapproval or even jail may be a price worth paying for the short-term benefits of a 'carefree' or 'normal' emotional and sexual relationship. In many cases, partners collude with or even instigate this assessment and, balancing the relative risks, decide that the maintenance of the relationship transcends the risk of HIV-transmission.

Our findings confirm the primacy of personal relationships in sexual risk-taking. This gives us some insight into how people with HIV deal with the sexual-social risk equation. Risk-taking is a common feature of sexual relationships: the risk of being emotionally or economically dependent, the risk of falling pregnant or contracting an STD, the risk of domestic violence, etc. Indeed, taking risks within relationships is part of a long cultural tradition in Western society in which we are all potentially 'fools for love'. Conjugal partnerships based on love are expected and idealized in Western tradition. The risk of HIV-transmission occurs within this cultural context; and PHAs balance it against other risks within relationships or the risk of having no relationship at all.

Notes

1   This section elaborates on findings previously reported in Sobo (1995b: Ch. 9) and Sobo (1997), with publishers' kind permissions.

2   At the time these data were collected, one of the husbands had recently died of AIDS; the other refused to be tested and may not actually have been infected.

3   Most talk of this strategy concerned casual sexual liaisons, but Maria also discussed non-disclosure conjoined with protective action in relation to her now-defunct IDU practice. She said, "I had already been positive when I got into the drug scene and [I was trying to not be] sharing needles and I used – I never said that I was HIV positive. The deal with it was I used, 'I'm a hemophiliac' – and then I found out you can't catch nothing from that! [laughter] And then I went through that I had hepatitis, and that, 'You will get sick from it [so] I don't share needles.' But I would not say I was HIV positive – I didn't want anybody to know. And this one guy insisted on taking my needle – insisting! I mean, he was ready to beat me up for this thing! Fine; good [sarcastically; i.e. how stupid]. And a long, long time I stood on that [excuse]. I never told him; I never told him [the truth]. But I also did tell him that he could get something. He still insisted on taking that syringe."

4   Maria remarked that she sometimes felt guilty for withholding serostatus information but, she said, in relation to one partner that she did not tell, "You know what? The guy turned out to be a real asshole anyway." Another time, a health care worker who had been fired and who knew the man that Maria was dating "told this guy that I was HIV positive. And the guy confronted me with it, and I denied it. I totally denied it, and he said, 'Well, if you had AIDS, you know, I would kill you'. ...But I never put him at risk."

5   At one point Eric also said, "Positive people shouldn't have sex with anyone." His view was exceptional.

6   On the other hand, because news of one's seropositivity has the potential to break a relationship up, being HIV positive can come in handy when a PHA decides that a relationship is not up to his or her standards, and feels comfortable with the possibility that information regarding his or her serostatus might become public knowledge. Timothy, an AIDS activist, did say, "I use it to get out of relationships sometimes." He also said, "I am not sure whether I use it to get into relationships [too]; that's one that I have been thinking about lately. I think it is very easy to kind of like – sometimes I analyse whether or not you use this kind of 'I am the poor victim' scenario as a way of getting the kind of people that I want to kind of like care for me."

7   Participants in a 1996 University College, London, Bloomsbury Medical Anthropology Seminar offered this hypothesis after being presented with the New Mexican data. Various scholars proposed (perhaps on the basis of a nationalistic bias) that the English had a larger sense of social responsibility and were less egocentric than US citizens.

8   Because of limitations in our methods, we cannot speculate on how widely held this model was among our gay participants. But we should point out that different guises of it may be quite common cross-culturally. It was even institutionalised in traditional Japan (Sobo 1987).

9 By this, he and the rest of the men generally meant that they chose partners 'wisely' (*cf.* Sobo 1993a, 1995b).

10 But one of those seven had a partner who already was seropositive. Only six experienced loving acceptance from seronegative or untested primary partners.

11 Much of this section elaborates on findings previously reported in Green (1994a; 1995c).

Chapter 11

Risk and reality:
the social situation

Both authors have heard many participants (as well as closer relations) lament the loss of members of their social networks since their seropositive diagnoses. And just over one-half (53%) of the Scottish PHAs reported having less contact with others since diagnosis, a change that they attributed to their HIV status. Intuitively, that such might happen would seem natural and inevitable, given the stigma associated with AIDS. However, as with much common-sense knowledge, until this hypothesis is tested, we will not be able to say for certain whether the pattern is real or perceived.

We know from the qualitative data presented in the preceding chapters that fears do not always pan out – although when they do it can be devastating. In this chapter, we examine quantitative social network data collected in Scotland that show that despite people's claims to have smaller and less supportive social circles as a result of being HIV positive, such does not seem to be the case across the board. We use qualitative data to explore the meanings of this quantitatively based finding, and we look to see if differences do emerge when we examine the data according to gender or lifestyle sub-category. A pattern perceived is no less significant than one that can be measured in terms of actual network shrinkage or reconfiguration, but the implications are of another order entirely.

HIV's effects on social support and networks: findings from the Scottish study

Social support

Our research in Glasgow involved not only PHAs but also a matched sample of seronegative individuals (for sample characteristics, see Table 4.2 in Chapter 4, p. 47). Both PHAs and seronegatives provided details regarding the composition of their social networks and social support.[1]

The social support scores of PHAs and seronegatives (see Table 11.1) were generally similar in all of the domains of social support that we measured. These included: social interaction, material support, and emotional support, which combined formed a total support score; confidant support; and stress resulting from support (Chapter 4 provided detailed explanations of these measures). The only significant difference found was that the PHAs perceived less available emotional support than the seronegatives did ($p<0.05$) and this difference is reflected in the marginally significant ($p<0.1$)[2] perception of total support available. Although there may have been no actual difference between the level of emotional support available to PHAs and seronegatives, it is equally plausible that the former may have felt more need for emotional support as a result of their diagnoses.

Network size

A comparison of the social contact and network composition of PHAs and seronegatives (see Table 11.2) reinforces the above social support findings. There was little difference in the average size of people's social networks, or in sociability (here defined as how often one meets with or talks to one's named social contacts). Nor were there marked statistical differences in the composition of social networks. For both PHAs and seronegatives, about one in ten of those persons named were household members; over one-half were non-resident kin; just under one-third were non-resident friends. There were no differences between PHAs and seronegatives with regard to whether they had a partner (about half did) or whether the partner was co-resident (about half were).

PHAs reported a greater number of contacts lost in the past year than seronegatives did. But this difference was not statistically significant. PHAs also named a slightly higher proportion of professional contacts as network members. But this was only a marginally significant difference ($p<0.1$).[3] It should, however, be noted that the sample size (66 PHAs and 67 seronegatives) was not large so that only

Table 11.1 Social support:[a] mean scores

	HIV+ (n = 66)	HIV– (n = 67)	F	Significance
Social interaction: mean scores and standard deviation				
Received	1.8 (0.5)	1.8 (0.4)	0.2	ns
Perceived	1.9 (0.4)	1.9 (0.4)	0.2	ns
Satisfaction with	0.7 (0.4)	0.7 (0.4)	0.0	ns
Material support: mean scores and standard deviation				
Received	0.6 (0.7)	0.7 (0.7)	0.7	ns
Perceived	1.6 (0.7)	1.7 (0.6)	0.3	ns
Satisfaction with	0.9 (0.3)	0.8 (0.3)	1.1	ns
Emotional support: mean scores and standard deviation				
Received	2.7 (1.3)	2.7 (1.0)	0.1	ns
Perceived	3.2 (1.1)	3.5 (0.8)	4.4	<0.05
Satisfaction with	0.8 (0.3)	0.8 (0.3)	0.5	ns
Total support: mean scores and standard deviation				
Received	5.0 (1.8)	5.2 (1.4)	0.5	ns
Perceived	6.7 (1.7)	7.1 (1.0)	3.1	<0.10
Satisfaction	0.8 (0.2)	0.7 (0.2)	0.4	ns
Support from confidants: mean scores and standard deviation				
Confidants	12.4 (4.2)	13.0 (3.6)	0.8	ns
Stress associated with social support: mean scores and standard deviation				
Stress	6.9 (4.0)	6.5 (3.7)	0.3	ns

a: For each measure a higher score = better support. The only exception is the score for stress associated with social support, where a higher score denotes greater stress.

quite marked differences between the two groups would be statistically significant. Non siginificant (ns) differences do not necessarily imply that there was no difference between the mean scores (see, for example, the scores for total persons in network, a difference that may have been statistically significant with a larger sample). Notwithstanding, in most measures, the social networks of PHAs and seronegatives were striking in their general similarity.

Disclosure's impact on social network membership

Seropositivity itself may not affect social network membership directly, at least when the PHA is asymptomatic. Self-disclosure, however, may have huge effects – or so common-sense knowledge would suggest. In order to ascertain more fully

Table 11.2 Social networks

Variable	HIV+ (n = 66) Mean (s.d.)	HIV– (n = 67) Mean (s.d.)	F	Significance
Sociability score	41.8 (16.9)	37.6 (15.5)	2.2	ns
Total persons in network	10.3 (3.4)	11.2 (3.3)	1.2	ns
Proportion household members	0.10 (0.14)	0.13 (0.14)	0.9	ns
Proportion non-resident kin	0.51 (0.21)	0.52 (0.17)	0.2	ns
Proportion non-resident friends	0.30 (0.20)	0.31 (0.19)	0.1	ns
Proportion professionals	0.09 (0.10)	0.05 (0.10)	2.8	<0.1
Number of lost contacts in last year	1.10 (1.4)	0.80 (1)	2.7	ns
Per cent (and no.) with no partner	50.0% (33)	49.3% (33)		ns
Per cent (and no.) with resident partner	25.8% (17)	22.4% (15)		ns
Per cent (and no.) with non-resident partner	24.2% (16)	28.4% (19)		ns

the significance of seropositivity for social network membership, we must ask how many members of the social network, and which members, were told about the diagnosis.

All but one participant in the Scottish study named at least one person in his or her social network that knew s/he was HIV positive. There were two participants however, who only named service workers as knowing.[4] It was rare for every listed member of the social network to know of the participant's diagnosis. Even those participants who had disclosed to the majority of network members sometimes chose not to disclose to one or two individuals who they felt either "would not be able to handle it" or "did not need to know." Children and grandparents often fell into these categories. Overall, however, 80 per cent of the Scottish sample members with HIV had more people in their networks that knew than did not know about their seropositive status. The mean per cent of network members who knew was 72 per cent.

About three-quarters (74%) of the 35 participants who were in contact with their fathers had disclosed their status to them, and two-thirds (66.6%) of the 48 who were in contact with their mothers disclosed to them. All but one of the 31 participants who had a long-term sexual partner at time of first interview had disclosed his or her status to that partner.

We found few differences in support by degree of disclosure. Those who told fewer people reported no more or less support than those who told many. But those who told more people had a greater number of PHAs in their social networks than those who told fewer people (p<0.05). The HIV-centredness of PHAs' networks seems a key variable.

Network HIV-centredness

Over 60 per cent of PHAs in the Scottish study included in their network someone they knew to be HIV positive and two participants listed five PHAs as close contacts. The mean number of other PHAs included in a social network was 1.1 – about one-tenth of a total network.

All PHAs knew at least one other HIV-positive person, although such persons were often very distant acquaintances. The mean number of PHAs known to them was 3.9. Over three-quarters knew or had known at least someone (often a friend of a friend who they had heard of but not necessarily met in person) who had AIDS; however, three men claimed to know over 20 such people directly (mean = 5.5; without these three, the mean = 4.4).

Most HIV-positive friends had been made as a direct result of a diagnosis. Health workers, for example, put one woman in touch with another HIV-positive woman, as both felt isolated. Some people, particularly many of the gay men, had met other PHAs in HIV support groups. Almost one-third (30.6%) had attended or were currently attending such a group.

Longitudinal data

Quantitative data about social networks and social support were collected from the PHAs at annual intervals over a three-year period (the seronegatives were interviewed once only). Analysis of the data revealed few changes in social interaction that could be related to HIV progression. There was some variation in the social support measures collected at times one, two and three but very few variations were statistically significant and no clear pattern could be identified. For example, the social support scores were somewhat lower a year after the initial interview, suggesting that perhaps support declines as the disease progresses, but this simple hypothesis was refuted the following year as support had increased to its baseline level.

An examination of the scores on a case-by-case basis showed that, of the eight PHAs whose health had clearly deteriorated during the three-year interview period, only three reported progressively less support at each interview; the remaining five reported few changes. In general, fluctuations over time in support and social networks among PHAs appeared to be related to life events such as being sent to or released from prison, or beginning or ending a long-term relationship.

Notwithstanding that networks remained much the same size throughout the study, there were a number of changes in their composition at each interview. Whether or not the networks of PHAs changed more rapidly than those of sero-negatives could not be measured as the latter were interviewed once only. There were, however, indications that the networks of PHAs were characterized by fairly rapid changes in network composition. The PHAs were slightly (although not significantly) more likely than seronegatives to report lost contacts and one-third became involved with HIV organizations after being diagnosed and they frequently made friends there.

Does gender make a difference?[5]

As more women in the economically developed world test HIV positive, the literature on the specific problems that women with HIV face also has grown (see Ilett's 1993 bibliography). Authors tend to focus upon issues that are clearly gender-linked, such as the natural history of HIV in women, female sexuality and motherhood, and women's differential access to, and needs from, health services (Bury *et al.* 1992; Corea 1992; Dorn *et al.* 1992; Sherr 1991; Doyal *et al.* 1994). It has been suggested that for women, particularly poor women, HIV is an essentially "different disease" than it is for men (Ward 1993a: 413).

Issues relating to the everyday social relationships of PHAs, however, are less clearly gendered and differences between men and women in this area have received little scholarly attention. Furthermore, the relationship between women and HIV is confounded by poverty (Farmer *et al.* 1993). Most women with HIV are from poor countries, or from poor and minority populations in more affluent ones, and they generally come from a background of poor physical and mental health, malnutrition, and inadequate medical care (Ward 1993a). So documented differences between men and women with HIV in terms of healthfulness and HIV's relation to social support may reflect the relative poverty of women rather than gender *per se*.

Findings point to few real gender differences (Quick *et al.* 1991), and women express overall satisfaction with support (Hankins 1993). However, lack of institutional support has been identified as a possible source of disadvantage for women (Crystal and Sambamoorthi 1996), and in recent years there has been a burgeoning of organizations world-wide offering such support specifically for women (Hankins 1993).

It is unclear whether women with HIV are more or less stigmatized than men although it is common for women with the virus to feel that they are seen as promiscuous or in some other or additional way socially deviant and irresponsible. This may be particularly the case among women who have injected drugs (Henderson 1992). Women with HIV in the developed world may be more prone to feel isolated (because, relative to men, fewer are infected) which may increase their feelings of stigma (Travers and Bennet 1996).[6]

Women's culturally idealized role as mother and homemaker may place those with HIV at a relationship-related disadvantage. Whilst children may decrease a woman's sense of isolation, there is the extra burden of concern about care for and eventual placement of children, disclosure of HIV status to them, and possible rejection by older children (Hankins 1993). It is also widely thought that women's relative powerlessness in sexual relationships may make disclosure of seropositivity to partners particularly traumatic (e.g. North and Rothenberg 1993).

We examined our Scottish social network data for quantitative evidence regarding the social relationships of men and women with HIV and their experiences of stigma. We use qualitative data to explore processes that may explain the quantitative results and to address issues such as women's child-care role. Although we do not have similar data for England or the USA, previously noted similarities in our data and similarities in the gender-related role expectations of each nation give strength to our supposition that the Scottish findings are generalizable.

Gender differences in social support and psychological well-being

Female PHAs listed more people in their social networks and had more contact with them than male PHAs.[7] As seen in Table 11.3, female PHAs scored higher than male PHAs on all measures of support, and most of the differences in male–female scores were statistically significant despite the small sample size. Indeed, on over half the measures, the differences were large enough to be statistically significant ($p<0.05$) in univariate and multivariate analysis (controlling for whether the participant was in prison, gay, had haemophilia or was currently injecting drugs).

Women reported significantly more social interaction than men ($p<0.01$), and more received and perceived support, and they were more satisfied with this support

Table 11.3 Mean (and standard deviation) for sociablility and social support scores by gender[a]

	Male (n = 54) Mean (s.d.)		Female (n = 12) Mean (s.d.)		Significance	Significance of indepen- dent effect
Total persons in network	9.9	(3.4)	12.1	(2.7)	0.05	0.001
Sociability score	39	(15.8)	53.9	(16.4)	<0.01	0.001
Total received support	5	(2.2)	6.5	(1.3)	<0.05	0.05
Total perceived support	7.3	(1.9)	8.7	(0.8)	<0.05	0.01
Total satisfaction with support	0.75	(0.24)	0.91	(0.1)	<0.05	0.01
Confidant support	11.8	(4.7)	4.1	(2.9)	ns	0.05
Stress connected with support	6.5	(3.7)	8.5	(4.4)	ns	0.10
Proportion living alone	60%		10%		0.01	0.01
Proportion with partner	40%		70%		ns	ns
Proportion with resident partner	20%		40%		ns	ns

a: For each measure a higher score = better support. The only exception is the score for stress associated with social support where a higher score denotes greater stress.

than were men (p<0.05). Significantly fewer of the women lived alone and more were partnered. The women reported slightly more support from confidants. Notwithstanding, they also reported more stress arising from their social relationships.

From these figures, it would seem that female PHAs were advantaged compared to male PHAs with regard to social interaction and social support. On average, they listed more people as important or close and had more frequent social interactions. From these interactions they also derived more support than the men. There were, however, few differences by gender with regard to the proportion of social network members who knew of the participant's HIV diagnosis.

Gender differences in HIV-related stigma

The female PHAs repeatedly claimed that the fact that AIDS was not associated in the public's mind with women made disclosing it harder for them than for men. But we found no evidence that women were less likely than men to disclose their serostatus to people in their social network – even to key people such as partners or parents. Nor were they less likely to know other PHAs. In this sense, women did not exhibit greater stigmatization or isolation in relation to disclosure frequencies *per se*.

Notwithstanding, perceptions of stigmatization were higher for women than men. In related research, carried out with a large proportion of the men and women who participated in the research described here, Green (1995a) found that women felt or perceived themselves to be more stigmatized than men. The female PHAs were more likely than the male PHAs to assess the attitudes of the general public to be hostile towards them.

The qualitative data we collected also suggested that women felt a greater sense of shame and stigma. In particular they felt tarnished by the 'dirty' image they felt others held of HIV, particularly its association with drug use and promiscuity.[8]

Women's home-based social role in Scotland also made them more visible and more vulnerable to stigma enacted by neighbours. Three of the 12 women in the Scottish study asked to be rehoused after neighbours "found out" about their HIV status, whereas only two of the 54 men reported being harassed by neighbours.

Child caring and rearing

Despite sometimes appalling victimization and stigmatization from strangers, neighbours or even health service workers, it was invariably stigmatizing responses from close friends and family that participants reported as most traumatic and hurtful. Whilst there were few gender differences in respect to the pain such incidents caused, being treated by close contacts as contaminating often occurred when a PHA came into contact with children (see Chapter 6). Therefore, women's childcare role made them particularly vulnerable to stigma from close contacts.

Over one-half (54.8%) of the Scottish PHAs (including one woman who had recently had a child) felt that PHAs should not have children, and 92.7 per cent estimated that this would be the attitude of the general public. They cited awareness of the transmission risk involved and the public opprobrium that would ensue. PHAs who want to conceive thus face enormous stigma (see Green 1995b).

Among the Scottish PHAs who brought up the subject of reproduction, we identified four groups based on attitudes to having children and life course stage. The first group (n = 9) reported that HIV had not been an issue for them in relation to reproduction since their diagnosis. They were over 30 and had children (many of whom were already young adults), and considered their families complete prior to diagnosis.

The second group (n = 10) was made up of single, childless PHAs in their early-to mid-twenties. They thought it unlikely that they would have children in the future and considered themselves ineligible as parents. Said Gina, "I couldn't think about bringing someone into the world and putting a life sentence on them. It's not fair."

Members of the third group (n = 8) were mostly in their late twenties and early thirties. All were partnered but none had children. They too thought it unlikely that they would have children in the future. For most this had nothing overtly to do with HIV: either they had never wanted children, or they thought that they were infertile. However, two in this group said that although they did not envisage parenting they hoped that medical advances would enable them to reproduce at a later date, if they so chose, without risk to partner or child.

The fourth group consisted of 12 participants (eight men and four women) who had either had a child since being diagnosed (n = 8), or had attempted to conceive or were thinking of doing so in the near future (n = 5).[9] It is of interest that the pregnancies when they occurred were always reported as an accidental consequence of contraceptive failure or as having happened before the respondent found out about their HIV-positive status. Whilst this may have been the case, it may also have been presented as such to minimise the blame and responsibility of potentially transmitting HIV to offspring, and therefore reducing the social risk. Members of this group were with one exception in their mid- to late thirties and had long-term partners (or did so when they conceived).

Stage in life course was clearly linked to attitudes about having children. For most participants, reproduction only became an issue when they settled into the sort of committed relationship in which they would normally be expected to reproduce. It was at this stage that pressure from partners or their commitment to the familial ideal might come to overshadow the fear of transmitting HIV to others.

Whilst decisions about reproduction clearly affected both men and women, given their role in gestation and in the family the issue was generally more pertinent to women than men. Three of the female participants were pregnant when diagnosed and two had attempted to conceive since diagnosis. All who wanted children had been strongly advised against it by the medical profession; Betty reported being sterilized against her will. All women who had borne a child after diagnosis reported highly stigmatizing hospital experiences at time of delivery. Said Heather, "The worst was when I had my daughter. I had to wait till I got home two days later to bath her. And every time they came in they had gloves on to pick her up."[10]

All the mothers in the sample were concerned about the stigmatization of their children. For example, Vicky moved out of her home when her neighbours found out about her HIV status and treated her son as contaminated. There was also much concern about disclosing to children for fear that they might talk about it at school and be victimized.

As noted in Chapter 6, both men and women reported stigmatization when they come into contact with children of friends and relatives. But perhaps due to gender expectations, all of the women in the sample raised this as a difficult issue whereas only about one-half of the men did. For women, contact with children was more of a day-to-day issue. For example, Heather reported that "my so-called best friend wouldn't let her kids come to my house" and Annie said, "My sister had her wee baby and she would not let me hold it." Such incidents fundamentally changed the nature of the participant's relationship with that person.

Equally offensive to participants were more covert expressions of child-related stigmatization. For instance, Keith said, "My wee nephew is a lovely wee boy and will come up and give you a hug. Now that has stopped. I have been told by my sister's husband he does not hug anybody anymore. [But he ...] hugs everybody else when they come in."

As Keith's testimony showed, contact with children was not exclusively a female practice, but in general the lifestyle of the women was more child-oriented compared to the men either in their role as mothers or child-minders, or due to the greater likelihood of their spending time with other mothers. Therefore, stigmatization in child-oriented contexts was more often directed at women. And the threat this posed to women in their role as child carers also meant that women felt the stigmatizing effects of such incidents more keenly.

Gender does make a difference

Disruption to social relationships and stigma affected both sexes and men and women faced similar issues and responses to disclosure. However, the impact of an HIV diagnosis varied according to gender and in relation to the different social roles that are ascribed to men and women. These social roles not only affected the contact points people had with AIDS stigma; they also affected the size and shape of people's social networks to begin with. Our findings thus support Ward's (1993a) observation that gender does make a difference.

Our findings showed that most women with HIV, like most women in the general population (Antonucci and Akiyama 1987; Turner and Marino 1994; Flaherty and Richman 1989; Schwarzer and Leppin 1988), and women with a chronic illness (Harrison *et al.* 1995), had larger and more supportive social networks than men. Good social support is generally perceived as beneficial to the mental health of PHAs (e.g. Hays *et al.* 1992, 1993). Despite the occasional disadvantage of a large support network, which might include increased stress and unwanted pressure, female PHAs were clearly advantaged in this respect.

With regard to HIV-related stigma, the women we talked with clearly felt more stigmatized than the men. The literature suggests that this may be a result of women's greater sense of isolation or because services for HIV tend to be oriented towards gay men (O'Sullivan and Thomson 1992). From the evidence presented here, however, social risk may be even more related to women's childbearing and child caring roles, which – at least in Western tradition[11] – are far more child-oriented than men's.

The impact of HIV upon social relationships was then gender distinct, and difference was rooted in gendered social roles. Family cohesion, social network maintenance, and caring for children tend to be female responsibilities, which helps us understand why women with HIV had more social support but felt more stigmatized than men. Whilst women's larger and more supportive social networks may indeed act as a buffer in coping psychologically with chronic illness (see Wortman 1984), the greater stigmatization felt by women with HIV may counteract this advantage.

Does lifestyle make a difference?

While the experience of being HIV positive was unique for each individual, some generalizations can be made. We saw above how the seropositive experience was, in some respects, different for men and women. Here, we examine differences according to lifestyle category. The term 'lifestyle category' is crude and putting individuals into groups that they might not necessarily define themselves as belonging to is problematic, but such categorization does enable us to make some comparisons and to identify some general trends.

The lifestyle groupings we use are: gay men, current injecting drug users (IDUs), people with haemophilia and, for statistical comparison, 'other' (a highly hetero-geneous group of eight women and eight men who were infected either through previous drug use, heterosexual activity, or contaminated blood).[12] Comparisons by ethnicity or race were impossible because all of the Scottish participants were non-Hispanic whites.[13]

We would not wish to suggest, however, that (for example) every gay male PHA's experience would fit the findings we present for gay male PHAs in general. Rather, we hope to demonstrate how who one is, in terms of defining social characteristics, affects the process of identity construction and the experience of being HIV positive.

Psychosocial variation by lifestyle

The psychosocial impact of an HIV diagnosis may vary according to social characteristics of sufferers. Both drug users and gay men belong to groups that have experienced social rejection and high levels of lifetime pathology (Catalan 1990), which may predispose those with the added burden of HIV to increased psychosocial distress. On the other hand, people with haemophilia have lived with chronic ill health all their lives, which may equip them well psychologically for coping with HIV (Wilkie *et al.* 1990).

The few studies comparing heterogeneous groups have tended to find that some PHAs and certain transmission groups are more vulnerable to psycho-social disorders than others. Psychopathological risk has been reported to be higher for seropositive gay men than drug users (Cazzullo *et al.* 1990). Fleishman and Fogel (1994) found avoidance coping and depressive symptoms to be more prevalent among members of disadvantaged groups in their seropositive sample: non-whites, drug users, women and those with lower incomes. Differences also have been found in the mental health of Black and white seropositive gay men. For example, Ostrow *et al.* (1991) found that Black gay US men with HIV were most reliant on their families for social support despite the fact that family members tended to disapprove of the gay identity and of 'having AIDS'. In contrast, the social support networks of white gay men were mostly composed of gay friends, who were more accepting of their condition (see also Wolcott *et al.* 1986; Namir *et al.* 1989a; Hays *et al.* 1990). Davis (1995) notes that white gay men in her study rated their spousal families more important sources of support while Blacks and Hispanics rated their biological families as more important sources.

Our data confirmed that, in some respects, coping with an HIV diagnosis varied according to social indicators. For example, the haemophiliacs appeared to cope well with the health implications of HIV. They reported being far less upset than other groups by hospital appointments as this was something they were already accustomed to. They were also used to taking medication and being restricted by illness. The older ones, who had lived with haemophilia before the widespread use of factor VIII[14] in the 1970s, had also experienced uncertain health (never knowing when a 'bleed' may become terminal) and a fairly short life expectancy. All the people with haemophilia reported that this had equipped them well for coping with the physiological aspects of HIV.

The multiple socio-economic problems of most IDUs, who made up another of our lifestyle categories, sometimes exacerbated problems associated with HIV but also tended to reduce its salience. HIV became one of many problems and was rarely the most important on a day-to-day level. For example, Betty was more concerned about her partner's domestic violence, Robbie about the welfare of his family while he was in prison, and Bill about finding money to pay the bills. John became aggressive when the interviewer repeated a question about the impact of HIV upon his life, insisting, "I keep telling you HIV makes nae [no] difference." These examples, all taken from the narratives of current IDUs, often had as much to do with general poverty as with drug use. The constant fear of being without food, housing, heating or adequate clothing reduced the impact of HIV on day-to-day life.

Social network and lifestyle

We looked for evidence in the Scottish sample of variability in social support by lifestyle category. Table 11.4 shows the mean scores for social support measures for people with haemophilia, current IDUs, gay men and others. Overall, gay men appeared to have the best social support networks, scoring highest on most measures and almost significantly higher than other groups for received support ($p < 0.1$).

People with haemophilia had the greatest number of social interactions, which reflected the family- or household-centredness of their networks: only one lived alone and all were either living with a long-term partner or with their parents. Nonetheless, they had the least received and perceived social support and fewer confidants than any other group. For received support, compared to other groups, they had significantly less ($p < 0.01$). But to rely on this figure alone as an index to their psycho-social health would be a mistake: other figures show that they were no less satisfied with their support, and experienced less stress from their support networks than did members of the other groups ($p < 0.05$). Also demonstrating the importance of viewing these figures holistically is the fact that the support networks of IDUs were similar to the other groups but the IDUs were significantly less satisfied with them ($p < 0.01$).

Table 11.4 Mean (and standard deviation) for sociability and social support scores by lifestyle category[a]

	Haemophiliac (n = 10)		Current drug user (n = 26)		Gay male (n = 14)		Other (n = 16)	
Network size	10.40	(4.1)	10.40	(3.3)	10.50	(3.1)	9.90	(3.4)
Sociability	46.30	(18.2)	40.98	(17.3)	43.80	(15.0)	38.14	(17.6)
Received support	3.30	(2.1)	5.70	(1.8)	6.40	(1.9)	5.00	(2.4)
Perceived support	6.80	(2.4)	7.30	(1.8)	8.60	(0.7)	7.60	(2.0)
Satisfaction	0.82	(0.2)	0.69	(0.3)	0.79	(0.2)	0.89	(0.1)
Confidant support	11.10	(4.2)	12.30	(3.9)	13.50	(4.5)	11.60	(5.5)
Stress	4.10	(3.1)	6.80	(3.8)	8.70	(3.6)	7.10	(4.1)

a: For each measure a higher score = better support. The only exception is the score for stress associated with social support, where a higher score denotes greater stress.

There were few differences by lifestyle category with regard to the proportion of the social network that knew of the participant's HIV status. There was a slight tendency for a greater proportion of the social networks of IDUs and gay men to know the participant was HIV positive, but these differences were not statistically significant. Overall, these findings point to no general conclusions about the variability of social support by lifestyle category.

It is clear, however, that people with haemophilia were far less likely than the others to include other PHAs in their social networks. Participants in general reported that about one in ten people in a network was also HIV positive, but for people with haemophilia the corresponding figure was one in 100 ($p<0.05$). There is thus evidence that the networks of people with haemophilia were less HIV-centred than the networks of members of the other groups.

Social risk and lifestyle

To illuminate the link between these findings and the social risk of an HIV identity, and to see how this social risk varies by lifestyle category, we examine once again the double stigma of AIDS. PHAs who belong to already stigmatized groups face a clear-cut double stigma. Further, people's attitudes about drug use, race, poverty, and homosexuality influence how they feel about interacting with PHAs (see Green 1995a). Non-drug-using PHAs thus have to contend with being labelled as 'junkies'; heterosexual PHAs may be assumed gay or 'promiscuous'. Thus all PHAs are doubly stigmatized whether or not they belong to an otherwise-stigmatized group.

Our data suggested that the double stigma affected most keenly those PHAs who did not belong to already stigmatized groups. In addition to them perceiving others' felt or expressed assumptions about their behaviour as incorrect, they were themselves often as homophobic and anti-IDU as many others in society. They thus found themselves ascribed a label that they abhorred, and the social risk associated with disclosure was consequently more pronounced for them. Disclosure carried the risk of shattering their social identity and disrupting their projected biographies.

A number of gay and drug-using participants found themselves similarly compromised, in that not all gay men were 'out' to all their social contacts (see Lang 1991), and many people injected drugs covertly. Such PHAs did, however, have the advantage of being accustomed to the stigma associated with gay sex and drug use. Prior to their HIV diagnosis, they had become experienced at managing a stigmatized identity. For those who openly incorporated the gay or IDU label as part of their identity already, HIV was more readily incorporated into their sense of self, conforming to the 'biographical enforcement' model put forward by Carricaburu and Pierret (1995).

Some may argue that those not belonging to stigmatized groups have a lower social risk as they are perceived as innocent and therefore targets for sympathy rather than hostility. Whilst sympathy may be forthcoming for children with HIV, our studies suggest that this was not in general the case for adults. They were not presumed innocent until proven guilty; rather, the opposite pattern prevailed.[15]

Public perception: voices from the streets

We began this chapter by examining the fact that, although the PHAs perceived shrinkage of network had occurred in response to their HIV diagnosis, there was no evidence that their networks were smaller than those of the seronegative controls. This suggested that PHAs' perception of the impact of HIV upon social networks was more dramatic than the reality of it. We now examine the match between PHAs' perception of public attitudes and those that the public actually professes to hold.

The severe social consequences accompanying an HIV-diagnosis were clearly expressed by all participants. For example, in separate interviews, Scottish participants John, Brian, and Michael talked about the stigma they had felt since receiving the HIV-positive diagnosis:

I've had less contact with people since my diagnosis. I've become more reserved with people and I walk about convinced that I have a stamp on my head: 'HIV'

The average person is ignorant about HIV like going back to leprosy and people being unclean and people seeing it with panic

I know a lot of moral society would be against me sleeping with anybody so I have guilt from that feeling

Similar statements run through the English and New Mexican transcripts.

These statements reflected participants' general feeling that public attitudes towards PHAs were quite negative, and that this exacerbated the negative effects of the disease on the social lives of PHAs. We have shown above that some of these effects were not as large as PHAs expected (which is not to say they were any less harmful or painful). But did the public really have such punitive attitudes towards PHAs? Did PHAs have an accurate assessment of public attitudes towards them? Did this assessment fit with the public's own perception of the attitudes of generalized others?

During the time our studies were conducted, the literature about public attitude to PHAs consistently suggested that the majority of people supported the rights of PHAs (e.g. Wellings and Wadsworth 1990) but that a minority of the population world-wide, normally about one-fifth, held very negative attitudes (Porter 1993; Ralston *et al.* 1992; Kunzel and Sadowsky 1993; Elliott *et al.* 1992; Dab *et al.* 1989; Peruga and Celentano 1993; Nisbet and McQueen 1993). Expressions of this hostility were described in Chapter 2.

We have seen in previous chapters, and in the social network data above, how PHAs incorporated and internalized negative standards attributed to the wider society and discredited themselves. Perceived social norms and related negative public attitudes towards PHAs were thus important sources of stigma. Accordingly, PHAs' perceptions of the attitudes of generalized others seemed to be a crucial indicator of felt stigma, and an over-estimation of the hostility of public attitudes would indicate a high level of felt stigma.

Green conducted a street survey in shopping areas in Scotland which aimed to measure (a) public attitudes to PHAs, and (b) the extent to which these differed, if at all, from PHAs' perceptions (see Green 1995a for full details). Participants in the street survey were asked to state what they thought themselves about PHAs, and what they thought that others thought about PHAs. People in a street survey may not always tell the truth, and in diverse areas, from smoking and drinking to racial discrimination, attitudes are not a very reliable indicator of behaviour (Fishbein 1967; La Piere 1934).[16] Notwithstanding, as Green also administered the street survey to the PHAs in the study this book describes, it provides a good comparative measure of the views of PHAs and those of the public they daily faced.

A quota sample of 300 adults stratified by gender, age, and location were asked to complete a 15-item questionnaire about attitudes to people with HIV. Interviews were conducted in 14 different locations in and around Glasgow and Edinburgh.[17] Participants were asked to rate 15 items describing views about people with HIV on a Likert-type scale ranging from 'strongly agree' to 'strongly disagree'. The street sample's self-reported attitudes were taken to represent the actual attitudes of 'the public'. The survey was also completed by 42 PHAs in the Scottish study during the second annual contact. In addition to providing their own views, all participants (the street sample and the PHAs) were asked to complete the questionnaire from the point of view of 'a typical member of the public'.

The street survey showed that, overall, the Scottish public had a relatively liberal view of PHAs and younger adults had more liberal attitudes than older adults. The majority felt that PHAs should expect some restriction on their freedom and should not bear children. The PHAs held somewhat more liberal attitudes than the street sample.

The most striking difference was between people's perceptions of others' attitudes and their own professed attitudes. PHAs attributed far more illiberal views to the public than the street sample reported, and so too did the street sample. There was a strong tendency among both PHAs and the street sample to overestimate the hostility of public attitudes.

Evidence of felt stigma among PHAs

While social desirability concerns may have biased people's presentation of themselves as more forgiving or liberal than others, these results provide evidence of felt stigma among PHAs. The disjunction between PHAs' own views and their perception of public attitudes was far greater than that of the street sample members, although the general belief that others were hostile toward PHAs was held by both groups.

The fact that the street sample as well as the PHAs apparently over-estimated the hostility of public attitudes suggested that the minority hostile viewpoint was believed to be the majority viewpoint. In other words, it was generally assumed that public attitudes were more hostile than they were, and in this sense the stigma related to HIV held by some appeared to have become generalized. This general-ization appears to have resulted from features of the illness (notably its infectious and as yet incurable nature and its association with already stigmatized groups), and processes such as media negativity and urban legend proliferation (as discussed in Chapter 2).

A shared hostile perception of the attitudes of others may have a different impact upon PHAs than those whose serostatus is negative or unknown. Whilst a member of the latter group may feel concerned and angry that others hold illiberal views, a PHA would surely feel stigmatized walking down a street thinking that most people view PHAs as dirty, different, guilty, weak and dangerous.

Are PHAs overestimating the odds of a bad reaction?

AIDS stigma was strongly felt by PHAs in all lifestyle categories and of each gender. We have heard testimony confirming that stigmatizing behaviour did occur and demonstrating the depth of victimization and humiliation PHAs were made to endure. Negative experiences were real and could be very damaging to self-esteem. They resulted in some people resisting assumption of an HIV-related identity and internalizing a sense of shame and unworthiness.

Why did some people resist while others did not? Why did some embrace HIV as an identity or identity component, and use their 'dangerousness' in a powerful and positive way (or reject it)? On the basis of the findings presented in this chapter we suspect that network strength and HIV-centredness has much to do with this. So too does membership in a gay community or a politically active one.

In addition to providing subjective testimony on what it feels like to be stigmatized as a PHA, we also have provided data demonstrating that feelings of stigmatization might not accurately reflect certain planes of social reality. Felt stigma may not correspond to the experience of stigma in an objective sense. It may have more to do with media hype and urban legends (which reach rural areas through the mass media and through social gossip chains). It may also have more to do with the cultural construction of the moral citizen than the real ways in which people live their lives. In the final chapter, we return to the question of identity and social risk.

Notes

1 This section elaborates on analysis reported in Green *et al.* (1996).
2 Statistical significance is denoted by a p value of <0.05. A value between >0.05 and <0.1 is defined as 'marginally significant'. A p value which is greater than 0.1 denotes a non-significant (ns) difference between the two groups.

3   That HIV-positive gay men had more professionals in their networks than seronegative gay men did was also found in a study in Australia (Packenham 1998).

4   Service workers were only included in the social network list if they met the criteria of having had frequent contact in the last month or who were important or particularly close to the respondent.

5   The section on gender draws heavily, and with kind publisher permission, upon Green (1996).

6   The women who set up the British organization 'Positive Women', for example, had difficulties locating other HIV-positive women (O'Sullivan and Thomson 1992).

7   No comparison was made between female PHAs and female seronegatives as the total number of women in the two samples combined (n = 24) was not large enough for meaningful statistical analysis.

8   Straight males also may feel isolated; Kevin, a straight Englishman said, "I have never met a straight person with HIV yet." When asked about self-diclosure, he told us, "In the gay community yes [people disclose to partners] but not in the straight community ... because it is still classed as a gay disease, it is a gay thing, it is nothing to do with heterosexuals it is homosexuals so if a straight lad thinks he has got it then [they think] he must have done something nutty."

9   One woman, who was diagnosed when pregnant and subsequently delivered a healthy child, had attempted to conceive again later on.

10 While this might have been for the baby's protection, the participant did not perceive it as such nor did it seem to have been explained to her by the staff as such.

11 There is some evidence that traditional gender role expectations are more strongly held by lower income and non-cosmopolitan individuals, and this research did concentrate on these populations.

12 Seven of the sample who had been infected as a result of injecting drugs had been free of drugs (including prescribed drugs) for at least a year before the interview, and were therefore deemed 'other'. Two participants believed they had been infected sexually but were using drugs at the time of the interview and they were placed in the 'IDU' category.

13 It should, however, be noted that there is some evidence of a marked difference between the social support networks of Black and white gay men in certain Western populations (see Ostrow *et al.* 1991; Leserman *et al.* 1992); the findings presented in this chapter may not apply to non-white populations in the Western world.

14 Factor concentrates such as Factor VIII are blood clotting agents which are widely used to prevent and stem 'bleeds' in people with haemophilia. Factor VIII's widespread use since the mid-1970s has revolutionized treatment, life expectancy and the quality of life for people with haemophilia.

15 The classification of some PHAs as 'innocent' perpetuates the belief that most PHAs are 'guilty' or have brought on their infections, and so we find it problematic.

16 La Piere (1934) toured the United States in the 1930s with a Chinese couple and stayed at 67 hotels and ate at 184 restaurants. In only 11 of these establishments did they receive less than average reception and they were only once refused service. Six months later a

questionnaire was sent to the same establishments asking if they would accept Chinese people as guests. Over 90 per cent of those who replied said that they would not. Although the divergence between attitude and behaviour in La Piere is the opposite of the divergence under discussion here, it serves to illustrate the enormous gap that may sometimes exist between behaviours and reported attitudes.

17 Interviews were conducted in six locations in Glasgow, one in a nearby suburb and one in a nearby town; and in six locations in Edinburgh. They were selected to give a broad range of types of areas in the two cities, e.g. central and peripheral shopping centres, high- and low-income residential areas including one where there was a high concentration of people with HIV.

Chapter 12

Seropositivity, identity, and social risk

Stigmatized selves

When asked about existing stereotypes of PHAs and the ways they might affect his sense of self, Jamie (England) told his interviewer, "I am sure you have read Susan Sontag. ...You should go away and read it." Sontag (1991) has described how certain diseases that are not well understood become imbued with negative meanings, and HIV in particular, due largely to its association with undesirable behaviour and its infectiousness, has been so imbued. For people diagnosed as HIV positive, these meanings can take on personal significance.

We have argued that self-construction is an ongoing process and that, in crafting and seeking to maintain certain kinds of selves, people largely seek to live up to the cultural expectations for personhood that they have internalized. A positive HIV diagnosis has the potential to shatter one's previously crafted sense of self because of the cultural connotations of AIDS and the practical consequences of being HIV positive. It also provides the individual with a potential new identity facet, one that s/he may integrate wholly, partially, or not at all, into a new sense of self.

As part of the process of renegotiating the self, PHAs can come to believe that they are indeed dirty, dangerous, and undesirable. This can happen as a result of stigmatizing reactions, especially when they come from health care workers (HCWs), who should be objective, or close social contacts, who should offer support. But, as

192

the following interchange with a Scottish participant shows, PHAs do not have to be told overtly that they are worthless or bad; they may internalize cultural stereotypes and assume the worst on their own.

Vanessa: I think aye there is still a stigma attached to it although people don't show it towards you.

GG: Where do you think that stigma comes from?

Vanessa: I think it really comes from inside you.

Shame, secrecy and the self-denial of supportive relationships

Because of a fear of stigma and unpleasantness in social interactions, many PHAs are wary of self-disclosure. Clearly, many PHAs do have negative self-disclosure experiences, as findings described in this book demonstrate. However, our data show also that networks need not shrink; in fact, some grow bigger and PHAs often grow closer to many of their social contacts. 'Authentic success' with self-disclosure was common, and although some participants reported bouts of delayed, hidden or tacit rejection ('inauthentic successes'), outright rejection was rare, particularly from sexual partners and close kin.

Our data show a clear gap between what PHAs believe about their social networks and what has actually happened to them in practice. The majority of PHAs in our studies expected most people to have hostile attitudes to PHAs and they expected that this hostility would be reflected by some of the people in their social networks. As a result they tended toward caution in disclosure to social contacts, although they were not always able to achieve this as their control over information about their HIV status sometimes was usurped by gossipers or HCWs.

The Scottish sample, for which we have specific social network data, tended to think that their social networks had shrunk substantially since diagnosis. They reported examples of rejection attributed to their HIV status, as did all the participants. In practice, however, Scottish social networks were relatively stable during the three-year study period. We have reason to believe that for New Mexico and North-East England, had we collected quantitative social network data, we would have seen more of the same.

How can we make sense of this gap between subjective perception and objective reality? Some PHAs in our studies clearly experienced very negative reactions to disclosure and some certainly lost friends as a result. Many of those who had not still had heard tales of others for whom this had been the case. These facts, in conjunction with the stigma associated with AIDS, in particular the felt stigma of PHAs, promoted an overly pessimistic assessment of the social risk entailed in disclosure to most people. In the eyes of many PHAs, the 'worst case scenario' of outright rejection became the norm and disclosure was a traumatic process thus confined to those who had a 'need to know'.

AIDS as a chronic illness

In his review of sociological research on chronic illness, Bury (1991) identifies two types of 'meaning' in chronic illness: the consequences for the individual (e.g. disruption of everyday life due to symptoms), and the cultural significance of illness (i.e. the connotations and imagery of the illness). Both types of meaning may affect how people see themselves and how they think others see them. Changes in symptoms and their disruptiveness further affect societal responses and these in turn will influence an individual's experience of his or her chronic illness state.

We have seen how people with HIV, like people with other chronic illnesses, confront not only the physical deterioration but also the negative meaning with which society imbues chronic illness. Our findings show that the cultural significance of AIDS has an extraordinary impact both on PHAs and society's reaction to them. This is not to deny that people with other chronic illnesses are not greatly affected by stigma too, but rather to highlight the fact that the stigma related to AIDS is similar to that of all chronic disease but at the same time it is very extreme. The double stigma of AIDS and the dramatic manner in which the disease first appeared has meant that AIDS has been viewed as something akin to a threatening alien intrusion and PHAs as dangerous intruders (recall the urban legends about AIDS discussed in Chapter 2; see also Farmer 1992; Sobo *et al.* 1997).

Like all chronic illness diagnoses, a diagnosis of HIV thus involves not just "biographical disruption" as described by Bury (1982: 167), and "disrupted feelings of fit" (Mathieson and Stam 1995: 293), but precipitates a "drama of identity construction" (Sandstrom 1990: 270). For AIDS represents both the danger from within and without, and the PHA is the ambivalent other, like a weed in a well-manicured garden. As such, an HIV-linked identity is one of the most socially risky identities in our society. This explains why so many PHAs prefer to keep this aspect of self hidden.

Notwithstanding, our findings suggest that, despite the identity work required, PHAs can and do carve out a meaningful sense of self, and with careful navigation of the risk landscape, can retain and build meaningful social relationships. Faced with such a monumental task, some PHAs have become instrumental in challenging the stigma associated with chronic illness in general and AIDS in particular.

PHAs such as Oscar Moore, who wrote a weekly column in *The Guardian* (a highly respected UK broadsheet) entitled 'Life as a PWA', have played a key role (see also Moore 1996). Moore was part of an on-going movement to demystify AIDS, promote the rights of PHAs, and campaign for more resources for fighting the disease. Those involved with this movement have exploited the high profile of AIDS, e.g. by distributing red ribbons, naming a World AIDS Day, and organizing rock concerts transmitted globally. Such initiatives aim to raise awareness of AIDS, and build solidarity with people affected by it throughout the world. This strategy, which has also been adopted by groups representing people with other chronic illnesses, has prompted a more general movement to lessen the social stigma and promote greater societal understanding of chronic illness.

Possible futures

Recommendations regarding self-disclosing in social settings

Although expressed opinions do not necessarily predict actual behaviour, evidence from this study suggests that people's attitudes to HIV may not be as punitive or stigmatizing as those infected, or the public, believe them to be. This finding merits attention, as reports from previous studies have tended to highlight the views of the illiberal minority rather than the liberal majority. Realization by PHAs that stereotypes about them may be held by a minority rather by everybody may help to lessen the felt stigma of an HIV diagnosis and underpin a more accurate assessment of social risk.

Moreover, there is some evidence that attitudes towards PHAs have become more liberal since the research described here was carried out. The *World AIDS Day 1997 News* (National AIDS Trust 1997) compares results of surveys undertaken by the UK Health Education Authority in 1989 and 1996. In 1989 over 50 per cent of those questioned agreed that PHAs had only themselves to blame and 36 per cent thought that employers should have the legal right to fire HIV-positive employees. On the other hand, 60 per cent thought PHAs got less understanding than they deserved. In 1996 the figures had changed to 36 per cent, 18 per cent, and 70 per cent respectively, demonstrating greater liberalization in attitudes to PHAs.

Similarly, negative attitudes in the USA have decreased over time (Herek and Glunt 1993) and this trend seems to be persisting.

There is also an increasing recognition of the effectiveness (in terms of prolonged life expectancy) of protease inhibitors and combination therapies. HIV infection is now compared more readily with other chronic rather than terminal disease states. Given that part of the stigma of HIV is due to its association with death, one would expect the longer life expectancy to result in a further liberalization of public attitudes. This largely depends, however, on whether the new therapies prove effective in the long term, and whether they become available to the majority of PHAs.

As we enter the new millennium, the ground would appear to be relatively fertile for a de-stigmatization of HIV disease. Public education campaigns need to emphasise the fact that PHAs can live relatively long and productive lives. They need to highlight the unjustness of ostracizing PHAs from areas of life in which they could fully participate with no risk of infection to others. This may help alleviate the felt stigma of an HIV diagnosis, and the undesirable effects on social relationships and psychological well being that may result from felt stigma.

Recommendations regarding public settings

Health care

As the rate of new infections with HIV has stabilized, and PHAs in UK and USA have increased life expectancy, panic in the health care arena has decreased and attitudes towards PHAs have softened. HCW organizations have issued guidelines about the treatment of PHAs, there are many specialist units treating PHAs, and HCWs have become more familiar with treating them. There is therefore every reason to suppose that enacted stigma towards PHAs in health care settings is becoming rarer, at least in areas where HIV prevalence is high. In time, this should lead to a decrease in felt stigma also, although it is likely that the time lag may be great. The memory of a harsh word from a HCW or being treated by a 'spaceman' lingers, and incidents several years old still loom large in the consciousness of many PHAs today.

Many HCWs have tried to provide a stigma-free environment for the health care of PHAs. It is important that they continue to seek ways of achieving this goal in order to encourage PHAs to attend for treatment, to feel comfortable about disclosure and to believe that HCWs do not see them as 'social lepers'. PHAs usually respect HCWs and look to members of the medical profession to maintain their health for as long as possible. Stigmatizing behaviour towards the patient with HIV threatens the relationship between HCW and patient, and the patient may respond by avoiding contact or by losing faith in the HCWs' competence to heal.

In the biomedical model of disease, stigma is not attached to disease and the reality of stigma may therefore be ignored or neglected by the medical profession (Williams 1987). It is clear that, at least in the 1980s, many HCWs were unaware of the extraordinary power of HIV-related stigma for shaping their interactions with PHAs. Many HCWs however gradually became aware of the social dimension of seropositivity when treating PHAs and through HIV-related training. Whilst this may have reduced the number of negative experiences PHAs have had in many health care settings, the declining publicity of and funds for HIV research may mean that many HCWs are now not acquiring experience or advice about appropriate social interaction with PHAs under their care (regarding AIDS complacency, see Feldman 1995; Singer 1999; Sobo 1999). It is essential that we continue to train HCWs in the social, personal and emotional dimensions of AIDS.

Health education and the production of stigma

So many AIDS programmes are oriented toward primary prevention, and biomedicine places so much emphasis on curative work, that there may be a tendency to feel that someone for whom HIV infection was not prevented has somehow failed to live by the standards that education campaigns set. PHAs can themselves internalize the belief that they have been their own undoing ("Don't die of ignorance" was a favoured UK AIDS education refrain). As Wang points out, "health promotion campaigns [may be] seen as potentially contributing to the production of stigma for people who already possess the attributes targeted for prevention" (1993: 77). Intervention planners and AIDS service workers of all types must not forget this; forethought must be given to the harmful consequences of programmes that "pathologize individuals as helpless, defective, and incapable of meeting their own needs" (p. 80). Sensitivity is called for in all aspects of service provision.

Recommendations regarding self-disclosing to sexual partners

Despite the fact that not all HIV-positive individuals self-disclose, particularly to casual or secondary sex partners, study findings support research indicating that many seropositive people do increase safer sex practices (e.g. Cleary *et al.* 1991; Schaefer *et al.* 1995). Further, findings support the conclusion that self-disclosure and safer sex are not the same thing; the former does not necessarily entail the latter (Perry *et al.* 1990b, 1994; Green 1995c). Safer sex must be promoted to HIV-positive individuals, their self-disclosure behaviours notwithstanding. Not only should sexual partners be protected, as with condoms, but the health of HIV-positive individuals themselves should be guarded through proactive efforts. The theme of self-protection that surfaced in participants' discourse could be exploited (in the USA, this centred around the common cold; in the UK, other strains of HIV and germs in general).

While safer sex is the best protection against infection, it is not foolproof. That is, even when safer sex is practised, HIV infection could possibly be spread. HIV-positive individuals must be informed and reminded of this. Such knowledge can encourage self-disclosure because it can increase the 'need to know' that the sero-positive individual will attribute to potential sex partners. Information regarding the mechanisms of denial among the seronegative (e.g. Sobo 1995b) also can encourage self-disclosure in this fashion. If PHAs are reminded that others often fail to internalize AIDS prevention knowledge, then they may not be so quick to accept an initial reluctance to practise safer sex on a partner's part as if an informed choice.

The HIV-related altruism indicated by the reported frequency with which the individuals in this study attempt beneficent prophylaxis is supported by other research, especially with women (Kline and VanLandingham 1994) but also with men (Solomon and DeJong 1989). This altruism could be tapped into as part of PHA counselling in regard to methods for persuading partners to take precautionary measures (see Taylor and Lourea 1992; Valdiserri *et al.* 1989; Vander Linden 1993).

Interventions also must be tailored to take into account whether individual clients may be pre-disposed to engage in risky sex. Recent community-based research[1] shows that predictors of continued high-risk sex include having higher numbers of male sex partners, a greater sense of physical well being, a poor relationship with one's physician, and a live-in sexual partner (Heckman *et al.* 1998).

Recommendations for counselling

Regarding the self-disclosure process, counsellors can encourage clients to test potential disclosees with strategic invitational advances. J. Green (1989b) encourages counsellors and clients to practise self-disclosing through role playing. It is important that clients sometimes play the role of the partner being disclosed to in order to gain at least some understanding of the feelings this may entail. If the situation warrants it, counsellors may point out that, as this research indicates, many people have self-disclosed with positive results. However, counsellors should prepare clients for possible future traumas by noting that rejection can lurk below superficial avowals of acceptance.

A further recommendation regarding counselling also can be made based on the findings. Participants from all sites recounted feeling confused or shocked after learning of a HIV-positive diagnosis. New PHAs seem to have trouble absorbing information provided in the post-test setting, a tendency noted by McCann and Wadsworth (1991).[2] For instance, although discussion of partner notification issues (as well as of other issues) was supposed to have occurred in post-test counselling for the New Mexicans, none recalled any such discussion. Partner notification must, therefore, be broached during later contact sessions as well. This means that great efforts must be taken to ensure future encounters with clients, who all too often, it seems, abandon counselling early on. In light of our findings, it may be most helpful for staff members interested in ensuring continued contact to make efforts to compensate for possible heightened sensitivity on clients' parts.

Flexible approaches to de-stigmatization

Gender differences have implications for service provision for PHAs, as men and women may require different kinds of support. Men, for example, especially straight men, or homosexuals not involved in a gay community, may have greater need of emotional support from services than women as women are more likely to have access to this type of support through their informal networks. But women may require more encouragement to contact HIV-related services due to the greater sense of felt stigma.

Provision of non-stigmatizing environments where women can feel at ease and bring their children would appear to be an important need for HIV-positive women. Assistance with child-care is also of enormous help for mothers with HIV, especially when they are ill or have to attend clinic appointments. During the time the fieldwork was carried out in Scotland, the following organizations catered to both men and women: Milestone House (a hospice and respite care centre for PHAs), SOLAS (a café and centre with courses for PHAs), and Positive Help (an organization which provides practical help such as babysitting for people affected by HIV). All were sensitive to gender issues and as a result attracted female PHAs as well as male PHAs and provided them with much needed support.

It is not just women with children who need to be made to feel welcome. Straight men also have reported problems, as have gay males and IDUs. And, as we have noted, PHAs may be hyper-vigilant in regard to stigmatizing experiences and this needs to be taken into account. In order to encourage clients to take full advantage of available counselling services, staff members should make special efforts to carry out duties as if these are elected tasks that have expressive or moral value. Clients who sense staff members' lack of commitment or tendency to lecture will turn away. This was noted mainly by the New Mexican participants; at the time of the research, their service organizations were mostly staffed by non-PHAs. Having PHAs in staff positions can be very helpful and should be encouraged, but cliquish behaviour among PHAs who serve staff functions is to be discouraged, as other PHAs who would seek services may feel shut out. A number of complaints regarding such were lodged against certain service organizations by participants in North-East England.

Where many bi- and homosexual men are served, offices and their staff should display gay-friendly attitudes, as by keeping up-to-date gay publications in waiting rooms. At the same time, if non-homosexual persons are to be served in the same centre, an effort must be made to make them feel welcome too.[3]

In short, when trying to appeal to clients, a range of variables need to be considered and a range of options made available. For example, PHAs living in relative deprivation may value benefit or welfare assistance advice far more than emotional support. Support agencies must recognize that HIV is only one part of a PHA's identity and the salience of the HIV will vary for each PHA accordingly, and very possibly over time, for each individual PHA. A flexible approach is therefore needed and we would urge all PHAs, their significant others, acquaintances and people PHAs come into contact with to behold the person behind the stigmatized identity and interact with that person rather than the HIV that, for some, that person has become.

Social risk and identity

Everyone is faced with the task of managing social risks. The risk may be related to aspects of identity such as having undesirable physical traits, or having been involved in previous misdemeanours, or being of a religious persuasion not typical among one's peers. Risks may also arise in unfamiliar or new social situations where rules of conduct are unknown, as when visiting a foreign country or participating in a ritual that one has never taken part in before. We are all aware of the potential dangers resulting from lack of cultural understanding by which a gesture of friendliness in one culture may mean quite the reverse in another.

The PHA, however, is faced with a particularly difficult task in social risk management as s/he carries one of the most stigmatizing conditions now known. Whilst many authors have written about the management of a stigmatized identity, and some have focused specifically upon HIV, in this book we have tried to reformulate the concept of stigma in terms of the sociology of risk. And we have done so from an anthropological perspective that highlights the cultural processes and models that we bring into play when dealing with friends, close kin, lovers, and other members of our social networks.

The narratives of PHAs regarding their management of social risk support Carter's (1996) assertion that identity is integral to risk perception and management. Each PHA's management of his or her perceived dangerousness is both fed by, and fed into, his or her sense of who s/he is; each designs his or her own unique style of risk management in relation to notions of self. Our data on PHAs' management of risk also show that even those labelled by society as dangerous and 'sick' or 'unhealthy' outsiders can and do construct their own version of the outsider, and portray themselves in contrast as morally respectable and therefore 'healthy' insiders. In other words, although some PHAs have been labelled as witches or monsters, even those most likely to be labelled as such can find persons more fitting the image to contrast themselves in good light against.

We can also see from the narratives of PHAs how social risk management operates within an individualized landscape of risk, and the way in which this landscape constantly changes as the components within it dance around each other (Adams 1995). Within this shifting landscape, individual PHAs at times engage in rationalist risk balancing exercises to make decisions about disclosure. For example, they organize their thoughts in terms of costs and benefits. Yet because risk-related decisions are intimately linked to the landscape of risk, a small change in the landscape may necessitate an entirely new set of calculations, or even negate the strategy of making carefully considered decisions to begin with. As such, risk-related equations couched in the economic idiom are rarely stable enough to be the sole basis of action. The interface between the individual's identity and the landscape of risk is constantly in motion, making risk behaviour an inherently dynamic and multiplex process.

Because our focus is specifically *social* risk we have not addressed the issue of health risk behaviours, such as drinking or smoking among PHAs. Had we done so, we believe we would have found a similar situation to that described for social risk behaviour: decisions are set against a dynamic, changing scenario of self and within the shifting landscape of risk. That is, some PHAs would opt for a healthy lifestlye to bolster their immune systems and others would choose the path of living dangerously on the grounds that they have to make the most of the short time left to them, or because all of their friends smoke and drink and they need to remain engaged in supportive social relations. Most PHAs, however, would probably carve a path that incorporated both ends of this spectrum, and at different times, as circumstances changed, veer to either one pole or the other. Risk management is a context-dependent process and it is complicated by the fact that it is contingent on yet another context-dependent process: that of identity construction and maintenance.

Identity and context are thus crucial ingredients in the management of social risk. Who one is, where one is, and who one is with largely determine one's perception and management of the social risk of being HIV positive, and dictate the extent to which HIV is incorporated publicly and privately into one's identity. And while certain facets of identity, such as gender, are fixed for almost everyone throughout life, other aspects may change over the life course (e.g. age, marital status, occupation).

Rapid and often temporary shifts in identity are not at all uncommon. Indeed, identity may change in an instant; recall the image of the prim librarian who, when the right man comes along, unbuttons her high-collared blouse, removes her austere glasses, unravels her severe bun, and becomes a pert and sexy good-time girl, ready for a night of love. While this hyperbolic image is part of a (rather sexist) myth, less calculated shifts in identity can occur frequently and rapidly, often requiring little more than a change of clothes. We each have many diverse (indeed, often contradictory) identities and the identity we choose or are forced to portray at one point in time may not be the same as the one preceding it or the one that will come after. This is all the more true when considering shifts in one's identity over the long-term, and under the influence of biographically salient experiences and incidents.

This is not to suggest that identity is superficial and simply changes to suit each situation. On the contrary, people do manage to build solidity into their private and public perception of who they are, largely because of relationships or other forms of biographical consistency (e.g. the reinforcement of certain aspects of one's self by close kin or through occupational expectations). A sense of self is also crafted through the use of cultural models of what de Munck calls "coherence mechanisms"; that is, salient ideas around which identity can coalesce (1992). But identity is malleable and multifaceted, and the self one chooses or is socially encouraged to portray is determined by a symbiotic relationship between who one thinks one is and the situation in which one finds oneself.

Social risk behaviour for people with HIV is dependent on the extent to which HIV is incorporated into identity. We have seen that this may vary according to illness stage and that those with visible symptoms of AIDS may have little option but to incorporate HIV, or at least the notion of being someone with a chronic illness, into their identity. Identity is not, after all necessarily freely chosen. Bill (Scotland), for example, was informed of his diagnosis in a prison cell with an open door in a voice loud enough for inmates in an adjoining room to hear. He had little option, at least while incarcerated, but to carry the identity of a person with HIV.

Those at an asymptomatic stage and whose HIV status has been handled more discreetly may prefer to keep HIV out of their public identity and sometimes they chose to keep it out of their private identity too. A small but consequential number of our respondents said that when first diagnosed they refused to believe the diagnosis and successfully convinced themselves that they were not HIV positive.

In addition to whether they have symptoms, the degree to which an HIV status is perceived or felt to be stigmatizing figures in people's HIV-identity decisions. Few of those with haemophilia or infected heterosexually told more than their very closest contacts (usually co-resident family and primary sexual partners) that they were PHAs, fearing the double stigma associated with the HIV label. This is not to suggest, however, that gay men or IDUs readily incorporated HIV into their identity. Whilst for some gay men the process was facilitated by their prior involvement with gay politics, few of the gay respondents were openly gay to all their social contacts. Likewise many IDUs preferred to keep their drug use private in some circumstances. In either case, self-identifying as a PHA would entail disclosures of gayness or of being an IDU, and so it could not happen.

We have seen that HIV disrupted some individuals' biographies more than others' and that for some people the diagnosis could even precipitate a form of what Carricaburu and Pierret (1995: 65) refer to as "biographical reinforcement". That is, while some people perceived their identity as spoiled by HIV as it precluded them from fulfilling their expected social roles, others were able to enfold it into their sense of self. This process is well illustrated by Mark and Eric (Scotsmen) who reported readily incorporating HIV into their identities. Mark was a gay man from a small village who had come to live in Glasgow following his diagnosis and quickly involved himself in self-help groups for PHAs. He found the process liberating and described his diagnosis as "one of the most positive things to have happened in my life". A number of people in the English and American samples reported similar activities and feelings of fulfilment. For Eric, on the other hand, HIV was compatible with the untamed biker image he aspired to prior to diagnosis.

Despite their primary embracement of their status as PHAs, at the time of interview Mark had still not told his family of his diagnosis, believing they would rather not know, and Eric had not told his employers, believing that he would lose his job if he did so. This illustrates the extent to which social context affects identity. Both men publicly embraced an HIV identity in most of the social settings in which they found themselves, but they preferred to downplay or ignore it in others (they also downplayed other aspects of self – gayness, biker lifestyle – in these other settings). The salience of social context was also apparent in earlier sections of this book, when we described the process of disclosure of HIV status in different settings, e.g. to acquaintances, friends, and family members (Chapters 6 and 7), health care workers (Chapter 8), and sexual contacts (Chapter 10). The disclosure strategies (and needs) of each individual varied from setting to setting.

An HIV-positive diagnosis carries with it high social risk and social uncertainty due to the dangers of being discriminated against, ostracized, rejected, or treated as 'spoiled'. One's management of this social risk and the degree to which HIV is incorporated into one's identity is dependent on one's perception of the likelihood of these problems occurring, and their significance.

In Chapter 3, we compared the process of disclosure decision-making to that of juggling a grand piano and a feather in a little boat on a turbulent sea. We think it fitting to return to this image to close, for the image brings to mind variety, irregularity, and constant motion. These words aptly describe the process of social risk management, even as it predictably follows the patterns we have described. Perhaps we also should provide our juggler with a host of different hats, to add to our moving picture constant (but unmeasured) shifts in his or her identity, like those that occur when people shift roles or experience changes in status throughout their lives. We do so now, to illustrate the uneven, ever-shifting, context-dependent nature of the individual, identity-linked process of managing social risk.

Notes

1   The study cited did not collect gender data but we can assume that both men and women answered the survey. Nonetheless, as the number of PHAs who are male is much greater than the number who are female, the gender-linked meaning of these findings should be interpreted with care.

2   McCann and Wadsworth (1991) studied the experience of testing in a clinic in which post-test counselling was the policy and found that two in five (41 per cent, n = 252) seropositive people did not remember receiving AIDS information when they received their test results. This "raises questions about how much can be achieved immediately after a test result is given" (p. 52), when testees' assimilation capacities may be minimal.

3   One heterosexual participant reported being accused of lying about his serostatus by service workers at one outreach office.

Bibliography

Abelove, H. 1994. The politics of the 'gay plague': AIDS as a U.S. ideology. In *Body Politics: Disease, Desire, and the Family,* M. Ryan and A. Gordon (eds), 3–17. San Francisco: Westview Press.

Ablon, J. 1981. Dwarfism and social identity: self-help group participation. *Social Science and Medicine* 15B, 25–30.

Ablon, J. 1995. 'The Elephant Man' as 'self' and 'other': the psycho-social costs of a misdiagnosis. *Social Science and Medicine* 40, 1481–1489.

Aboulafia, D.M. 1998. Occupational exposure to human immunodeficiency virus: what healthcare providers should know. *Cancer Pract* 6, 310–317.

Adam, B. and A. Sears 1994. Negotiating sexual relationships after testing HIV-positive. *Medical Anthropology* 16, 63–77.

Adam, B. and A. Sears 1996. *Experiencing HIV.* New York: Columbia University Press.

Adam, B. 1998. *Timescapes of Modernity: The Environment and Invisible Hazards.* London: Routledge.

Adams, J. 1995. *Risk.* London: University College London Press.

Albrecht, G.L., V.G. Walker and J.A. Levy 1982. Social distance from the stigmatized: a test of two theories. *Social Science and Medicine* 16, 1319–1327.

Alonzo, A.A. and N.R. Reynolds 1995. Stigma, HIV and AIDS: an exploration and elaboration of a stigma trajectory. *Social Science and Medicine* 41, 303–315.

Anderson, R. and M. Bury 1988. *Living With Chronic Illness: The Experience of Patients and Their Families.* London: Unwin Hyman.

Anon 1992. AIDS in the family. *British Medical Journal* 304, 1639–1640.

Antonucci, T.C. and H. Akiyama 1987. An examination of sex differences in social support among older men and women. *Sex Roles* 17, 737–749.

Ariss, R.M. with G.W. Dowsett 1997. *Against Death: The Practice of Living with AIDS.* Amsterdam: Gordon and Breach.

Arnston, P. 1986. The perceived psycho social consequences of having epilepsy. In *Psychopathology in Epilepsy: Social Dimensions,* S. Whitman and B. Hermann (eds). Oxford: Oxford University Press.

BIBLIOGRAPHY

Bailey, F.G. 1983. *The Tactical Uses of Passion: An Essay on Power, Reason, and Reality.* Ithaca, NY: Cornell University Press.

Balshem, M. 1993. *Cancer in the Community: Class and Medical Authority.* Washington DC: Smithsonian Institution Press.

Baltimore Sun. 1993. Women with AIDS risk assault by partners. October 14, 16A.

Barroso, J. 1997. Reconstructing my life: becoming a long-term survivor of AIDS. *Qualitative Health Research* 7, 57–74.

Bauman, Z. 1991. *Modernity and Ambivalence.* Cambridge: Polity Press.

Bauman, Z. 1992. *Intimations of postmodernity.* London: Routledge.

Beck, U. 1992. *Risk Society: Towards a new Modernity.* London: Sage.

Becker, H.S. 1963. *Outsiders: Studies in the Sociology of Deviance.* New York: Free Press.

Beharrell, P. 1993. AIDS and the British press. In *Getting the Message,* J. Eldridge (ed), 210–242. London: Routledge.

Bellaby, P. 1990. To risk or not to risk? Uses and limitations of Mary Douglas on risk acceptability for understanding health and safety at work and road accidents. *The Sociological Review* 38, 465–483.

Bender, D. and D. Ewbank 1994. The focus group as a tool for health research: issues in design and analysis. *Health Transition Review* 4, 63–80.

Bennet, M.J. 1990. Stigmatization: experiences of persons with acquired immune deficiency syndrome. *Issues in Mental Health Nursing* 11, 141.

Berrios, D.C., N. Hearst, T.J. Coates, R. Stall, E.S. Hudes, H. Turner, R. Eversley and J. Catania 1993. HIV antibody testing among those at risk for infection: the national AIDS behavioral surveys. *Journal of the American Medical Association* 270, 1576–1580.

Bloom, J.R. and L. Kessler 1994. Emotional support following cancer: a test of the stigma and social activity hypotheses. *Journal of Health and Social Behavior* 35, 118–133.

Bloom, J.R. and D. Spiegel 1984. The relationship of two dimensions of social support to the psychological well-being and social functioning of women with advanced breast cancer. *Social Science and Medicine* 19, 831–837.

Bloor, M. 1995a. A user's guide to contrasting theories of HIV-related risk behaviour. In *Medicine, Health and Risk: Sociological Approaches,* J. Gabe (ed), 19–30. Oxford: Blackwell Publishers Ltd.

Bloor, M. 1995b. *The Sociology of HIV Transmission.* London: Sage.

Bolton, R. and M. Singer (eds) 1992b. *Rethinking AIDS Prevention: Cultural Approaches.* Philadelphia: Gordon and Breach.

Bolton, R. and M. Singer. 1992a. Rethinking HIV prevention: critical assessments of the content and delivery of AIDS risk-reduction messages. In *Rethinking AIDS Prevention,* R. Bolton and M. Singer (eds), 1–5. New York: Gordon and Breach Science Publishers.

Bolton, R. 1992. AIDS and promiscuity: muddles in the models. In *Rethinking AIDS Prevention,* R. Bolton and M. Singer (eds), 7–85. New York: Gordon and Breach Science Publishers.

Bor, R., R. Miller and H. Salt 1991. Uptake of HIV testing following counseling. *Sexual and Marital Therapy* 6, 25–28.

Borchert, J. and C.A. Rickabaugh 1995. When illness is perceived as controllable: the effects of gender and mode of transmission on AIDS-related stigma. *Sex Roles* 33, 657–668.

206

Borden, W. 1991. Beneficial outcomes in adjustment to HIV seropositivity. *Social Service Review* 65, 434–449.

Brendstrup, E. and K. Schmidt 1990. Homosexual and bisexual men's coping with the AIDS epidemic: qualitative interviews with 10 non-HIV tested homosexual and bisexual men. *Social Science and Medicine* 60, 713–720.

Brook, L. 1988. The public's response to AIDS. In *British Social Attitudes the 5th Report*, R. Jowell, S. Witherspoon and L. Brook (eds), 71–91. Aldershot: Gower Publishing Company.

Brown, G.R. and J.R. Rundell 1993. A prospective study of psychiatric aspects of early HIV disease in women. *General Hospital Psychiatry* 15, 139–147.

Bury, J., V. Morrison and S. McLachlan (eds) 1992. *Working with Women and AIDS: Medical, Social and Counselling Issues*. London: Tavistock Routledge.

Bury, M. 1982. Chronic illness as biographical disruption. *Sociology of Health and Illness* 4, 167–182.

Bury, M. 1991. The sociology of chronic illness: a review of research and prospects. *Sociology of Health and Illness* 13, 451–468.

Cajetan Luna, G. 1997. *Youths Living with HIV: Self-Evident Truths*. New York: Harrington Park Press.

Cancian, F. 1987. *Love in America: Gender and Self-Development*. New York: Cambridge University Press.

Carricaburu, D. and J. Pierret 1995. From biographical disruption to biographical reinforcement: the case of HIV-positive men. *Sociology of Health and Illness* 17, 65–88.

Carter, S. 1995. Boundaries of danger and uncertainty: an analysis of the technological culture of risk assessment. In *Medicine, Health and Risk: Sociological Approaches*, J. Gabe (ed), 133–150. Oxford: Blackwell Publishers Ltd.

Carter, S. 1996. Reducing AIDS risk: a case of mistaken identity? *Science as Culture* 6, 220–245.

Catalan, J. 1990. Psychiatric manifestations of HIV disease. *Bailliere's Clinical Gastroenterology* 4, 547–562.

Catalan, J., I. Klimes, A. Bond, A. Day, A. Garrod and C. Rizza 1992a. The psychosocial impact of HIV infection in men with haemophilia: controlled investigation and factors associated with psychiatric morbidity. *Journal of Psychosomatic Research* 36, 409–416.

Catalan, J., I. Klimes, A. Day, A. Garrod, A. Bond and J. Gallwey 1992b. The psychosocial impact of HIV infection in gay men: a controlled investigation and factors associated with psychiatric morbidity. *British Journal of Psychiatry* 161, 774–778.

Cazzullo, C.L., C. Gala, S. Martini, A. Pergami, M. Rossini and R. Russo 1990. Psychopathologic features among drug addicts and homosexuals with HIV infection. *International Journal of Psychiatry in Medicine* 20, 285–292.

CDC [Centers for Disease Control and Prevention] 1998. *HIV/AIDS Surveillance Report* 10.

Charmaz, K. 1983. Loss of self: a fundamental form of suffering in the chronically ill. *Sociology of Health and Illness* 5, 168–195.

Chiodo, G. and S. Tolle 1992. A challenge to doctor-patient confidentiality: When HIV-positive patients refuse disclosure to spouses. *Dental Ethics* 40, 275–277.

BIBLIOGRAPHY

Cleary, P., N.V. Devanter, T. Rogers, E. Singer, R. Shipton-Levy, F. Steilen, A. Stuart, J. Avorn and J. Pindyck 1991. Behavior changes after notification of HIV infection. *American Journal of Public Health* 8, 1586–1590.

Cleary, P.D., M. Fahs, W. McMullen, G. Fulop, J. Strain, H. Sacks, C. Muller, M. Foley and E. Stein 1992. Using patient reports to assess hospital treatment of persons with AIDS: a pilot study. *AIDS Care* 4, 325–332.

Coates, T., R. Stall, S. Kegeles, B. Lo, S.F. Morin, L. McKusick 1988. AIDS antibody testing: will it stop the AIDS epidemic? Will it help people infected with HIV? *American Psychologist* 11, 859–864.

Conrad, P. 1987. The experience of illness: recent and new directions. *Research in the Sociology of Health Care* 6, 1–31.

Converse, P.E. 1964. The nature of belief systems in mass publics. In *Ideology and Discontent*, D.E. Apter (ed.). New York: The Free Press.

Corbin, J.M. and A. Strauss 1988. *Unending Work and Care: Managing Chronic Illness at Home*. San Francisco: Jossey-Bass.

Corea, G. 1992. *The Invisible Epidemic: The Story of Women and AIDS*. New York: Harper Collins.

Cote, T.R., R.J. Biggar and A.L. Dannenberg 1992. Risk of suicide among persons with AIDS. *Journal of the American Medical Association* 268, 2066–2068.

Cowles, K.V. and B.L. Rodgers 1997. Struggling to keep on top: meeting the everyday challenges of AIDS. *Qualitative Health Research* 7, 98–120.

Coyle, S.L., R.F. Boruch and C.F. Turner (eds) 1991. *Evaluating AIDS Prevention Programs* (Expanded edn). Washington DC: National Academy Press.

Crandall, C.S. and R. Coleman 1992. AIDS-related stigmatization and the disruption of social relationships. *Journal of Social and Personal Relationships* 9, 163–177.

Crandall, C.S. and D. Moriarty 1995. Physical illness stigma and social rejection. *British Journal of Social Psychology* 34, 67–83.

Crandall, C.S., J. Glor and T.W. Britt 1997. AIDS-related stigmatization: instrumental and symbolic attitudes. *Journal of Applied Social Psychology* 27, 95–123.

Crawford, R. 1994. The boundaries of the self and the unhealthy other: reflections on health, culture and AIDS. *Social Science and Medicine* 38, 1347–1365.

Crocker, J., B. Cornwell and B. Major 1993. The stigma of overweight: affective consequences of attributional ambiguity. *Journal of Personality and Social Psychology* 64, 60–70.

Crossley, M.L. 1997. 'Survivors' and 'victims': long-term HIV positive individuals and the ethos of self-empowerment. *Social Science and Medicine* 45, 1863–1873.

Crowther, M. 1992. I am a person, not a disease: experiences of people living with HIV/ AIDS. *Professional Nurse* March, 381–385.

Crystal, S. and U. Sambamoorthi 1996. Care needs and access to care among women living with HIV. In *AIDS as a Gender Issue: Psychosocial Perspectives*, L. Sherr, C. Hankins and L. Bennett (eds), 191–196. London: Taylor and Francis.

Dab, W., J.P. Moatti, S. Bastide, L. Abenhaim and J. Brunet 1989. Misconception about transmission of AIDS and attitudes towards prevention in the French general public. *AIDS* 3, 43–47.

Dalton, H. 1989. AIDS in blackface. *Deadalus* 118, 205–227.

D'Andrade, R. 1992. Schemas and motivation. In *Human Motives and Cultural Models*, R. D'Andrade and C. Strauss (eds), 23–44. New York: Cambridge University Press.

Davies, M.L. 1997. Shattered assumptions: time and the experience of long-term HIV positivity. *Social Science and Medicine* 44, 561–571.

Davis, F. 1964. Deviance disavowal: the management of strained interaction by the visibly handicapped. In *The Other Side*, H. Becker (ed), 119–138. New York: Free Press.

Davis, R.L. 1995. The casual influence of perceived quality of life on social support among HIV-positive individuals. PhD dissertation, University of California at Los Angeles.

Davison, C. 1991. Half-hearted about semi-skimmed. *Horizon* BBC TV, 24 June.

Davison, C., G. Davey Smith and S. Frankel 1991. Lay epidemiology and the prevention paradox. *Sociology of Health and Illness* 13, 1–19.

De Jong, W. 1980. The stigma of obesity: the consequences of naive assumptions concerning the causes of physical deviance. *Journal of Health and Social Behavior* 21, 75–87.

de Munck, V. 1992. The fallacy of the misplaced self: gender relations and the construction of multiple selves among Sri Lankan Muslims. *Ethos* 20, 167–189.

Dew, M.A., J. Becker, J. Sanchez, R. Caladararo, O.L. Lopez, J. Wess, S.K. Dorst and G. Banks 1997. Prevalence and predictors of depressive, anxiety and substance use disorders in HIV-infected and uninfected men: a longitudinal evaluation. *Psychological Medicine* 27, 395–409.

Dickson, G.C.A. 1991. *Risk Analysis*. London: Witherby and Co.

Dorn, W., S. Henderson and N. South (eds) 1992. *AIDS: Women, Drugs and Social Care*. London: Falmer Press.

Douglas, M. 1966. *Purity and Danger: an Analysis of Concepts of Pollution and Taboo*. London: Routledge and Kegan Paul.

Douglas, M. 1970. *Natural Symbols. Explorations in Cosmology*. Harmondsworth: Penguin.

Douglas, M. 1986. *Risk Acceptability According to the Social Sciences*. London: Routledge and Kegan Paul.

Douglas, M. 1990. Risk as a forensic resource. *Daedalus* 119, 1–16.

Douglas, M. 1992. *Risk and Blame: Essays in Cultural Theory*. London: Routledge.

Douglas, M. and A. Wildavsky 1982. *Risk and Culture: An Essay on the Selection of Technological and Environmental Dangers*. Berkeley: University of California Press.

Doyal, L., J. Naidoo and T. Wilton (eds) 1994. *AIDS: Setting a Feminist Agenda*. London: Taylor and Francis.

Dublin, S., P.S. Rosenberg and J.J. Goedert 1992. Patterns and predictors of high-risk sexual behavior in female partners of HIV-infected men with hemophilia. *AIDS* 6, 475–482.

Dunbar, S. and S. Rehm 1992. On visibility: AIDS, deception by patients, and the responsibility of the doctor. *Journal of Medical Ethics* 18, 180–185.

Dworkin, J., G. Albrecht and J. Cooksey 1991. Concern about AIDS among hospital physicians, nurses and social workers. *Social Science and Medicine* 33, 239–248.

Earl, W.L., C.J. Martindale and D. Cohn 1991–92. Adjustment: denial in the styles of coping with HIV infection. *Omega* 24, 35–47.

BIBLIOGRAPHY

Eich, D., A. Dobler-Mikola and R. Luthy 1990. Is quality of life associated with a specific risk behaviour in HIV-positive individuals? Paper (abstract SB376) presented at the VIth International Conference on AIDS, San Francisco.

Elliott, L., S. Parida and L. Gruer 1992. Differences in HIV-related knowledge and attitudes between Caucasian and 'Asian' men in Glasgow. *AIDS Care* 4, 389–393.

Ellis, S.J. 1993. Hysteria over doctors with HIV. *Lancet* 341, 764.

Ericson, R.V. and K.D. Haggerty 1997. *Policing the Risk Society*. Oxford: Clarendon Press.

Farmer, P. 1992. *AIDS and Accusation: Haiti and the Geography of Blame*. Berkeley: University of California Press.

Farmer, P., S. Lindenbaum and M.J. Delvecchio Good 1993. Women, poverty and AIDS: an introduction. *Culture, Medicine and Psychiatry* 17, 387–397.

Feldman, M. 1995. Attitude adjustment: a complacent public tunes out the AIDS epidemic. *Minnesota Medicine* 78, 10–14 and 64–65.

Fell, M., S. Newman, M. Herns, P. Durrance, H. Manji, S. Connolly, R. McAllister, I. Weller and M. Harrison 1993. Mood and psychiatric disturbance in HIV and AIDS: changes over time. *British Journal of Psychiatry* 162, 604–610.

Fischhoff, B., S. Lichtenstein, P. Slovic, S.L. Derby and R.L. Keeney 1984. *Acceptable Risk*. Cambridge: Cambridge University Press.

Fishbein, M. 1967. Attitude and the prediction of behavior. In *Readings in Attitude Theory and Measurement*, M. Fishbein (ed), 477–492. New York: John Wiley and Sons.

Fisher, J., K.K. Willcutts, S. Misovich and B. Weinstein 1998. Dynamics of sexual risk behavior in HIV-infected men who have sex with men. *AIDS and Behavior* 2, 101–113.

Fitzsimons, D., V. Hardy and K. Tolley 1995. *The Economic and Social Impact of AIDS in Europe*. London: Cassell.

Flaherty, J. and J. Richman 1989. Gender differences in the perception and utilization of social support: theoretical perspectives and an empirical test. *Social Science and Medicine* 28, 1221–1228.

Fleishman, J.A. and B. Fogel 1994. Coping and depressive symptoms among people with AIDS. *Health Psychology* 13, 156–169.

Frankenberg, R. 1994. The impact of HIV/AIDS on concepts relating to risk and culture within British community epidemiology: candidates or targets for prevention? *Social Science and Medicine* 38, 1325–1335.

Frazer, J.G. 1979 [1890]. Sympathetic magic. In *Reader in Comparative Religion: An Anthropological Approach*, W. Lessa and E. Vogt (eds), 337–352. San Francisco: Harper and Row.

Freeman, M. 1993. *Rewriting the Self: History, Memory, Narrative*. London: Routledge.

Gabe, J. (ed) 1995. *Medicine, Health and Risk: Sociological Approaches*. Oxford: Blackwell Publishers Ltd.

Gallop, R.M., G. Taerk, W. Lancee, R. Coates, M. Fanning and M. Keatings 1991. Knowledge, attitudes and concerns of hospital staff about AIDS. *Canadian Journal of Public Health* 82, 409–412.

Gard, L. 1990. Patient disclosure of human immunodeficiency virus (HIV) status to parents clinical considerations. *Professional Psychology: Research and Practice* 21, 252–256.

Gatter, P.N. 1995. Anthropology, HIV and contingent identities. *Social Science and Medicine* 41, 1523–1533.

Giddens, A. 1990. *The Consequences of Modernity*. Cambridge: Polity Press.

Giddens, A. 1991. *Modernity and Self-Identity*. Cambridge: Polity Press.

Giesecke, J., K. Ramstedt, F. Granath, T. Ripa, G. Rado and M. Westrell 1991. Efficacy of partner notification for HIV infection. *The Lancet* 338, 1096–1099.

Gifford, S. 1986. The meaning of lumps: a case study of the ambiguities of Risk. *In Anthropology and Epidemiology: Interdisciplinary Approaches to the Study of Health and Disease*. In C.R. Janes, R. Stall, S.M. Gifford (eds), 213–246. Dordrecht: Reidel

Glaser, B.G. and A.L. Strauss 1968a. *A Time for Dying*. Chicago: Aldine.

Glaser, B.G. and A.L. Strauss 1968b. *The Discovery of Grounded Theory: Strategies for Qualitative Research*. London: Weidenfield and Nicolson.

Glick-Schiller, N. 1992. What's wrong with this picture: the hegemonic construction of culture in AIDS research in the United States. *Medical Anthropology Quarterly* 6, 237–254.

Goffman, E. 1963. *Stigma: Notes on the Management of Spoiled Identity*. Englewood Cliffs, NJ: Prentice-Hall.

Gordon, D.R. 1990. Embodying illness, embodying cancer. *Culture, Medicine and Psychiatry* 14, 275–297.

Green, G. 1993. Editorial review: social support and HIV. *AIDS Care* 5(1), 87–104.

Green, G. 1994a. Positive sex: the sexual relationships of a cohort of men and women following an HIV-positive diagnosis. In *AIDS: Foundations for the Future*, P. Aggleton, P. Davies and G. Hart (eds), 136–146. London: Falmer Press.

Green, G. 1994b. The reproductive careers of a cohort of men and women following an HIV-positive diagnosis. *Journal of Biosocial Science* 26, 409–415.

Green, G. 1995a. Attitudes towards people with HIV: are they as stigmatising as people with HIV think they are? *Social Science and Medicine* 41, 557–568.

Green, G. 1995b. Processes of stigmatisation and impact on the employment of people with HIV. In *The Economic and Social Impact of AIDS in Europe*, D. Fitzsimons, V. Hardy and K. Tolley (eds), 251–262. London: Cassell.

Green, G. 1995c. Sex, love and seropositivity: balancing the risks. In *AIDS: Safety, Sexuality and Risk*, P. Aggleton, P. Davies and G. Hart (eds), 144–158. London: Taylor and Francis.

Green, G. 1996. Stigma and the social relationships of people with HIV: does gender make a difference? In *AIDS as a Gender Issue: Psychosocial Perspectives*, L. Sherr, C. Hankins, L. Bennett (eds), 46–63. London: Taylor and Francis.

Green, G. and S. Platt 1997. Fear and loathing in health care settings reported by people with HIV. *Sociology of Health and Illness* 19, 70–92.

Green, G., S. Platt, S. Eley and S.T. Green 1996. 'Now and again it really hits me': the impact of an HIV-positive diagnosis upon psychosocial well-being. *Journal of Health Psychology* 1, 125–141.

Green, J. 1989a. Counselling for HIV infection and AIDS: the past and the future. *AIDS Care* 1, 5–10.

Green, J. 1989b. Post-test counselling. In *Counselling in HIV Infection and AIDS*, J. Green and A. McCreaner (eds), 28–68. Boston: Blackwell Scientific Publications.

BIBLIOGRAPHY

Grinyer, A. 1995. Risk, the real world and naïve sociology. In *Medicine, Health and Risk: Sociological Approaches*, J. Gabe (ed), 31–52. Oxford: Blackwell Publishers Ltd.

Grove, K.A., D.P. Kelly and J. Liu 1997. 'But nice girls don't get it': women, symbolic capital, and the social construction of AIDS. *Journal of Contemporary Ethnography* 26, 317–337.

Handwerker, P. 1993. Gender power differences may be STD risk factors for the next generation. *Journal of Women's Health* 2, 301–316.

Hankins, C. 1993. Berlin Conference review – Women and AIDS: psychosocial issues. *AIDS Care* 5, 471–478.

Harrison, D., K. Wambach and J. Byers 1991. AIDS knowledge and risk behaviors among culturally diverse women. *AIDS Education and Prevention* 3, 79–89.

Harrison, J., P. Maguire and C. Pitceathly 1995. Confiding in crisis: gender differences in pattern of confiding among cancer patients. *Social Science and Medicine* 41, 1255–1260.

Hart, G. and M. Boulton 1995. Sexual behaviour in gay men: towards a sociology of risk. In *AIDS: Safety, Sexuality and Risk*, P. Aggleton, P. Davies and G. Hart (eds), 55–67. London: Taylor and Francis.

Hart, G., R. Fitzpatrick, J. Dawson, J. McLean and M. Boulton 1992. What's your excuse for relapsing? A critique of recent sexual behaviour studies of gay men. In *Private Risks and Public Dangers, Explorations in Sociology*, S. Scott, G. Williams, S. Platt and H. Thomas (eds), 133–149. London: Avebury.

Hassin, J. 1994. Living a responsible life: the impact of AIDS on the social identity of intravenous drug users. *Social Science and Medicine* 39, 391–400.

Hays, R.B., S. Chauncey and L. Tobey 1990. The social support networks of gay men with AIDS. *Journal of Community Psychology* 18, 374–385.

Hays, R.B., L. McKusick, L. Pollack, R. Hilliard, C. Hoff and T. Coates 1993. Disclosing HIV seropositivity to significant others. *AIDS* 7, 425–431.

Hays, R.B., R. Magee and S. Chauncey 1994. Identifying helpful and unhelpful behaviours of loved ones: the PWA's perspective. *AIDS Care* 6, 379–392.

Hays, R.B., H. Turner and T.J. Coates 1992. Social support, AIDS-related symptoms, and depression among gay men, *Journal of Consulting and Clinical Psychology* 60, 463–469.

Heckman, T., J. Kelly and A. Somlai 1998. Predictors of continued high-risk sexual behavior in a community sample of persons living with HIV/AIDS. *AIDS and Behavior* 2, 127–135.

Henderson, S. 1992. Living with the virus: perspectives from HIV-positive women's needs in Edinburgh. In *AIDS: Women, Drugs and Social Care*, W. Dorn, S. Henderson and N. South (eds), 8–29. London: Falmer Press.

Herek, G.M. 1990. Illness, stigma, and AIDS. In *Psychological Aspects of Serious Illness: Chronic Conditions, Fatal Diseases, and Clinical Care*, P.T. Costa Jr. and G.R. Vanden Bos (eds), 107–150. Washington DC: American Psychological Association.

Herek, G.M. 1997. The HIV epidemic and public attitudes toward lesbians and gay men. In *In Changing Times: Gay Men and Lesbians Encounter HIV/AIDS*, M.P. Levine, P.M. Nardi and J.H. Gagnon (eds), 191–218. Chicago: University of Chicago Press.

212

Herek, G.M. and E. Glunt 1988. An epidemic of stigma: public reactions to AIDS. *American Psychologist* 43, 886–891.

Herek, G.M. and E. Glunt 1993. Public attitudes toward AIDS-related issues in the United States. In *The Social Psychology of HIV Infection*, J.B. Pryor and G.D. Reeder (eds), 229–261. Hillsdale, NJ: Lawrence Erlbaum Associates, Inc.

Herek, G.M. and J.P. Capitanio 1998. Symbolic prejudice of fear of infection? A functional analysis of AIDS-related stigma among heterosexual adults. *Basic and Applied Social Psychology* 20, 230–241.

Herzlich, C. and J. Pierret 1987. *Illness and Self in Society*. Baltimore: The Johns Hopkins University Press.

Holland, J., C. Ramazanoglu, S. Scott, S. Sharp and R. Thomson 1990. Sex, gender and power: young women's sexuality in the shadow of AIDS. *Sociology of Health and Illness* 12, 336–350.

Holt, R., P. Court, K. Vedhara, K. Nott, J. Holmes and M. Snow 1998. The role of disclosure in coping with HIV infection. *AIDS Care* 10, 49–60.

Holtgrave, D., R. Valdiserri, A. Gerber and A. Hinman 1993. Human immunodeficiency virus counseling, testing, referral, and partner notification services. In *Archives of Internal Medicine* 153, 1225–1230.

Hood, C. and D.K. Jones (eds) 1996. *Accident and Design: Contemporary Debates in Risk Management*. London: University College London Press.

Hospital Infection Society and the Surgical Infection Study Group 1992. Risks to surgeons and patients from HIV and hepatitis: guidelines on precautions and management of exposure to blood or body fluids. *British Medical Journal* 305, 1337–1343.

Horsman, J.M and P. Sheeran 1995. Health care workers and HIV/AIDS: a critical review of the literature. *Social Science and Medicine* 41(11), 1535–1657.

Howarth, G. 1993. AIDS and undertakers: the business of risk management. *Critical Public Health* 4(3), 47–53.

Huby, G. 1999. Contesting 'needs': entitlement to welfare benefits for people with HIV/AIDS in Lothian, Scotland. *Anthropology and Medicine* 6, 143–152.

Hughes, E.C. 1945. Dilemmas and contradictions of status. *American Journal of Sociology* 50, 353.

Hutchinson, J. 1993. Delayed diagnosis of HIV/AIDS among women in the United States: its causes and health repercussions. Unpublished paper, Texas: University of Houston.

Ilett, R. 1993. *Women and HIV/AIDS – a Bibliograpy*. Glasgow: Glasgow Women's Library.

Ingham, R., A. Woodcock and K. Stenner 1991. Getting to know you...: young people's knowledge of their partners at first intercourse. *Journal of Community and Applied Psychology* 1, 117–132.

Jacoby, A. 1994. Felt versus enacted stigma: a concept revisited – evidence from a study of people with epilepsy in remission. *Social Science and Medicine* 38, 269–274.

Jemmott, L. and J. Jemmott 1991. Applying the theory of reasoned action to AIDS risk behavior: condom use among Black women. *Nursing Research* 40, 228–234.

Johnstone, F., L. Maccallum and R. Riddell 1990. Contraceptive use in HIV infected women. *British Journal of Family Planning* 16, 106–108.

Jones, E.E., A. Farina, A. Hastorf, H. Markus, D. Miller, R. Scott, and R. French 1984. *Social Stigma: the Psychology of Marked Relationships*. New York: W.H. Freeman and Company.

Joseph, J., R. Kessler and C. Wortman 1989. Are there psychological costs associated with changes in behavior to reduce AIDS risk? In *Primary Prevention of AIDS: Psychological Approaches*, V. Mays, G. Albee and S. Schneider (eds), 209–224. Newbury Park, CA: Sage Publications.

Kagawa-Singer, M. 1993. Redefining health: living with cancer. *Social Science and Medicine* 37, 295–304.

Kalichman, S. and J. Fisher 1998. Introduction to the special issue on risk-behavior practices of men and women living with HIV-AIDS. *AIDS and Behavior* 2, 87–88.

Kane, S. 1994. Criminal law on the heels of epidemiology: the arrest and sentencing of HIV-infected street prostitutes. Paper presented to the Annual Meetings of American Society of Criminology, Miami, November 9–12.

Kaufert, P.A. and J. O'Neill 1993. Analysis of a dialogue on risks in childbirth: clinicians, epidemiologists and Inuit women. In *Knowledge, Power and Practice: the Anthropology of Medicine of Everyday Life*, S. Lindebaum and M. Lock (eds), 32–54. Berkeley: University of California Press.

Kegeles, S., J. Catania and T. Coates 1988. Intentions to Communicate Positive HIV-Antibody Status to Sex Partners. *Journal of the American Medical Association* 259, 216–217.

Kegeles, S., T. Coates, T. Christopher and J. Lazarus 1989. Perceptions of AIDS: the continuing saga of AIDS-related stigma. *AIDS* 3 (Suppl. 1), S253–S258.

Kelly, B., B. Raphael, F. Judd, M. Perdices, G. Kernutt, G.D. Burrows, P.C. Burnett and M. Dunne 1998. Psychiatric disorder in HIV infection. *Australian and New Zealand Journal of Psychiatry* 32, 441–453.

Kessler, R.C., K. O'Brien, J.G. Joseph, D. Ostrow, J.P. Phair, J.S. Chmiel, C.B. Wortman and C.A. Emmons 1988. Effects of HIV infection, perceived health and clinical status on a cohort at risk for AIDS. *Social Science and Medicine* 27, 569–578.

King, M.B. 1989. Prejudice and AIDS: the views and experiences of people with HIV infection. *AIDS Care* 1, 137–143.

Kinsey, K. 1994. 'But I Know My Man': HIV/AIDS Risk Appraisals and Heuristical Reasoning Patterns Among Childbearing Women. *Holistic Nurse Practitioner* 8, 79–88.

Kitzinger, J. 1993. Understanding AIDS: researching audience perceptions of acquired immune deficiency syndrome. In *Getting the Message,* J. Eldridge (ed), 271–304. London: Routledge.

Kleinman, A. and J. Kleinman 1996. The appeal of experience; the dismay of images: cultural appropriations of suffering in our times. *Daedalus* 125, 1–23.

Klepinger, D.H., J.O. Billy, K. Tanfer and W.R. Grady 1993. Perceptions of AIDS risk and severity and their association with risk-related behavior among US men. *Family Planning Perspectives* 25, 74–82.

Kline, A. and M. VanLandingham 1994. HIV-infected women and sexual risk reduction: the relevance of existing models of behavioral change. *AIDS Education and Prevention* 6, 390–402.

Klitzman, R. 1997. *BeingPositive: The Lives of Men and Women with HIV*. Chicago: Ivan R. Dee.

Knudson-Cooper, M.S. 1981. Adjustment to visible stigma: the case of the severely burned. *Social Science and Medicine* 15B, 31–44.

Kowalewski, M.R. 1988. Double stigma and boundary maintenance: how gay men deal with AIDS. *Journal of Contemporary Ethnography* 17, 211–228.

Kubler-Ross, E. 1992. *On Death and Dying*. London: Routledge.

Kunzel, C. and D. Sadowsky 1993. Predicting dentists' perceived occupational risk for HIV infection, *Social Science and Medicine* 36, 1579–1584.

Kurth, A. and M. Hutchinson 1989. A context for HIV testing in pregnancy. *Journal of Nurse-Midwifery* 34, 259–265.

La Piere, R.T. 1934. Attitudes versus actions. *Social Forces* 13, 230–237.

Lancet 1991. Partner notification for preventing HIV infection. Vol. 338, 1112–1113.

Landis, S., V. Schoenbach, D. Weber, M. Mittal, B. Krishan, K. Lewis and G. Koch 1992. Results of a randomized trial of partner notification in cases of HIV infection in North Carolina. *New England Journal of Medicine* 326, 101–106.

Lang, N.G. 1991. Stigma, self-esteem, and depression: psycho-social responses to risk of AIDS. *Human Organization* 50, 66–72.

Laryea, M. and L. Gien 1993. The impact of HIV-positive diagnosis on the individual, part 1: stigma, rejection, and loneliness. *Clinical Nursing Research* 2, 245–266.

Laurenceau, J.P., L. Barrett and P. Pietromonaco 1998. Intimacy as an interpersonal process: the importance of self-disclosure, partner disclosure, and perceived partner responsiveness in interpersonal exchanges. *Journal of Personality and Social Psychology* 74, 1238–1251.

Lawless, S., S. Kippax and J. Crawford 1996. Dirty, diseased, and undeserving: the positioning of HIV positive women. *Social Science and Medicine* 43, 1371–1377.

Leserman, J., D.O. Perkins and D.L. Evans 1992. Coping with the threat of AIDS: the role of social support. *American Journal of Psychiatry* 149, 1514–1520.

Levi, J. 1996. Rethinking HIV counseling and testing. *AIDS and Public Policy Journal* 11, 164–168.

Limandri, B. 1989. Disclosure of stigmatizing conditions: the discloser's perspective. *Archives of Psychiatric Nursing* 3, 69–78.

Lindenbaum, S. and M. Lock (eds) 1993. *Knowledge, Power and Practice: The Anthropology of Medicine and Everyday Life*. Los Angeles: University of California Press.

Lindsay, M., H. Peterson and T. Feng 1989. Routine antepartum human immunodeficiency virus infection screening in an inner-city population. *Obstetrics and Gynecology* 74, 289–294.

Locker, D. 1983. *Disability and Disadvantage: The Consequences of Chronic Illness*. London: Tavistock.

Loustaunau, M. and E. Sobo 1997. *The Cultural Context of Health, Illness, and Medicine*. Westport, CT: Bergin and Garvey.

Lupton, D. 1993. Risk as moral danger: the social and political functions of risk discourse in public health. *International Journal of Health Services* 23, 425–435.

215

BIBLIOGRAPHY

Lupton, D. 1995. *The Imperative of Health: Public Health and the Regulated Body*. London: Sage Publications.

Lupton, D., S. McCarthy and S. Chapman 1995. 'Doing the right thing': the symbolic meanings and experiences of having an HIV antibody test. *Social Science and Medicine* 41, 173–180.

MacIntyre, A. 1985. *After Virtue*. London: Duckworth.

Mansergh, G., G. Marks and J.M. Simoni 1995. Self-disclosure of HIV infection among men who vary in time since seropositive diagnosis and symptomatic status. *AIDS* 9, 639–644.

Marks, G., J. Richardson and N. Maldonado 1991. Self-disclosure of HIV infection to sexual partners. *American Journal of Public Health* 81, 1321–1322.

Marks, G., N. Bundek, J. Richardson, M. Ruiz, N. Maldonado and H. Mason 1992a. Self-disclosure of HIV infection: preliminary results from a sample of Hispanic men. *Health Psychology* 11, 300–306.

Marks, G., J. Richardson, M. Ruiz and N. Maldonado 1992b. HIV-infected men's practices in notifying past sexual partners of infection risk. *Public Health Reports* 107, 100–106.

Martin, J.L. and L.L. Dean 1988. The impact of AIDS on gay men: a research instrument. Unpublished questionnaire, Columbia University, New York.

Marzuk, P.M., H. Tierney, K. Tardiff, E.M. Gross, E.B. Morgan M.A. Hsu and J.J. Mann 1988. Increased risk of suicide in persons with AIDS. *Journal of the American Medical Association* 259, 1333–1337.

Marzuk, P.M. and S.W. Perry 1993. Suicide and HIV: researchers and clinicians beware. *AIDS Care*, 5, 387–390.

Mason, H.R.C., G. Marks, J.M. Simoni, M.S. Ruiz and J.L. Richardson 1995. Culturally sanctioned secrets? Latino men's nondisclosure of HIV infection to family, friends, and lovers. *Health Psychology* 14, 1–7.

Mathieson, C.M. and H.J. Stam 1995. Renegotiating identity: cancer narrative. *Sociology of Health and Illness* 17, 283–306.

McCain, N.L. and L.F. Gramling 1992. Living with dying: coping with HIV disease. *Issues in Mental Health Nursing* 13, 271–284.

McCann, K. and E. Wadsworth 1991. The experience of having a positive HIV antibody test. *AIDS Care* 3, 43–53.

McCrystal, C. 1995. A town in turmoil, a church in crisis. *Observer* October 9, 19.

McGarrahan, P. 1994. *Transcending AIDS: Nurses and HIV Patients in New York City*. Philadelphia: University of Pennsylvania Press.

McKeganey, N. and M. Barnard 1992. *AIDS, Drugs and Sexual Risk: Lives in the Balance*. Milton Keynes: Open University Press.

McManus, J. 1994. *AIDS in the North: the Local Authority Perspective*. North of England Assembly of Local Authorities.

McQuillan, G., M. Khare, T. Ezzati-Rice, J. Karon, C. Schable and R. Murphy 1994. The seroepidemiology of human immunodeficiency virus in the United States household population: NHANES III, 1988–91. *Journal of Acquired Immune Deficiency Syndrome* 7, 1195–1201.

Meadows, J., S. Jenkinson and J. Catalan 1990. Voluntary HIV testing in the antenatal clinic: differing uptake rates for individual counselling midwives. *AIDS Care* 2, 229–233.

Miller, D. 1987. *Living with AIDS and HIV*. Basingstoke: Macmillan Press.

Moore, O. 1996. *Looking AIDS in the Face*. London: Pan Macmillan.

Morin, M., Y. Obadia, J.P. Moatti and M. Souville 1995. Commitment, value conflicts and role strains among French GPs in care for HIV positive patients. *AIDS Care*, 7(Suppl. 1), S79–S84.

Murphy, R.F. 1998. The damaged self. In *Understanding and Applying Medical Anthropology*, P.J. Brown (ed), 322–333. Mountain View, CA: Mayfield.

Namir, S., M.J. Alumbaugh, F. Fawzy and D.L. Wolcott 1989a. The relationship of social support to physical and psychological aspects of AIDS. *Psychology and Health* 3, 77–86.

Namir, S., D.L. Wolcott and F. Fawzy 1989b. Social support and HIV spectrum disease: clinical research perspectives. *Psychiatric Medicine* 7, 97–105.

National AIDS Trust 1997. *World AIDS day news*. London: National AIDS Trust.

Nation's Health. 1993. APHA fights criminalization of HIV exposure in Illlinois court. *Nation's Health* 23, 9.

Nisbet, M and D. McQueen 1993. Anti-permissive attitudes to lifestyles associated with AIDS. *Social Science and Medicine* 36, 893–901.

New Mexico HIV Disease Update 1994. 861 AIDS cases reported by 12/31/93. *New Mexico HIV Disease Update*. Division of Epidemiology, Evaluation and Planning, New Mexico Department of Public Health.

North, R and K. Rothenberg 1993. Partner notification and the threat of domestic violence against women with HIV infection. *New England Journal of Medicine* 629, 1194–1196.

Oliver, M. 1990. *The politics of disablement*. London: Macmillan.

Ostrow, D.G., A. Monjan, J. Joseph, M. Vanraden, R. Fox, L. Kingsley, J. Dudley and J. Phair 1989. HIV-related symptoms and psychological functioning in a cohort of homosexual men. *American Journal of Psychiatry* 146, 737–742.

Ostrow, D., R. Whitaker, K. Frasier, C. Cohen, J. Wan, C. Frank and E. Fisher 1991. Racial differences in social support and mental health in men with HIV infection: a pilot study. *AIDS Care* 3, 55–62.

O'Sullivan, S. and K. Thomson (eds) 1992.*Positively Women: Living with AIDS*. London: Sheba Feminist Press.

Packenham, K.I. (1998) Specification of social support behaviours and network dimensions along the HIV continuum for gay men. *Patient Education and Counselling* 34, 137–157.

Parsons, E. and P. Atkinson 1992. Lay constructions of genetic risk. *Sociology of Health and Illness* 14, 437–455.

Perkins, D.O., E.J. Davidson, J. Leserman, D. Liao and D.L. Evans 1993. Personality disorder in patients infected with HIV: a controlled study with implications for clinical care. *American Journal of Psychiatry* 150, 309–315.

Perry, S. and B. Fishman 1993. Depression and HIV. How does one affect the other? *Journal of the American Medical Association* 270, 2609–2610.

BIBLIOGRAPHY

Perry, S., C. Card, M. Moffatt, T. Ashman, B. Fishman and L. Jacobsberg. 1994. Self-disclosure of HIV infection to sexual partners after repeated counseling. *AIDS Education and Prevention* 6, 403–411.

Perry, S., L. Jacobsberg , B. Fishman 1990a. Psychological responses to serological testing for HIV. *AIDS* 4, 145–152.

Perry, S., J. Ryan, K. Fogel, B. Fishman and L. Jacobsberg. 1990b. Voluntarily informing others of positive HIV test results: patterns of notification by infected gay men. *Hospital and Community Psychiatry* 41, 549–551.

Peruga, A. and D. Celentano 1993. Correlates of AIDS knowledge in samples of the general population. *Social Science and Medicine* 36, 509–524.

Peterson, A. and D. Lupton 1996. *The New Public Health: Health and Self in the Age of Risk.* London: Sage.

PHLS [Public Health Laboratory Service] AIDS Centre 1998. United Kingdom: data to end September 1998 (Quarterly tables reported on the Website www.phls.co.uk). Accessed April 1999.

Pivnick, A. 1993. HIV Infection and the meaning of condoms. *Culture, Medicine, and Psychiatry* 17, 431–453.

Platt, S. 1992. Suicidal ideation and behaviour in human immuno-deficiency virus (HIV) disease, *Epidemiologia E Psichiatria Sociale* 1, 11–13.

Porter, S.B. 1993. Public knowledge and attitudes about AIDS among adults in Calcutta, India. *AIDS Care* 5, 169–176.

Powell-Cope, G. and M. Brown 1992. Going public as an AIDS family caregiver. *Social Science and Medicine* 34, 571–580.

Pryor, J.B. and G.D. Reeder. 1993. Collective and individual representations of HIV/AIDS stigma. In *The Social Psychology of HIV Infection,* J.B. Pryor and G.D. Reeder (eds), 263–286. Hillsdale, NJ: Lawrence Erlbaum Associates, Inc.

Pryor, J., G. Reeder, R. Vinacco and T. Kott 1989. The instrumental and symbolic functions of attitudes toward person with AIDS. *Journal of Applied Social Psychology* 19, 377–404.

Quick, P., M. Rees-Newton, I. Mackie and J. Gilmour 1991. Characteristics of men and women with HIV disease: a comparison of psychosocial issues. Paper presented at the VII International Conference on AIDS, Florence.

Quimby, E. 1992. Anthropological witnessing for African-Americans: power, responsibility, and choice in the age of AIDS. In *The Time of AIDS: Social Analysis, Theory, and Method,* G. Herdt and S. Lindenbaum (eds), 159–184. Newbury Park, CA: Sage Publications.

Quinn, N. and D. Holland. 1987. Culture and cognition. In *Cultural Models in Language and Thought,* D. Holland and N. Quinn (eds), 3–40. Cambridge: Cambridge University Press.

Rabkin, J.G., R. Goetz, R. Remien, J.B. Williams, G. Todak and J.M. Gorman 1997. Stability of mood despite HIV illness progression in a group of homosexual men. *American Journal of Psychiatry* 154, 231–238.

Rabkin, J.G., R. Remien, L. Katoff and J.B. Williams 1993. Suicidality in AIDS long-term survivors. *AIDS Care* 5, 401–411.

BIBLIOGRAPHY

Rabkin, J.G., J.B. Williams, R. Remien, R. Goetz, R. Kertzner and J.M. Gorman 1991. Depression, distress, lymphocyte subsets, and human immunodeficiency virus symptoms on two occasions in HIV-positive men. *Archive General Psychiatry* 48, 111–119.

Ralston, G., M. Dow and B. Rothwell 1992. Knowledge of AIDS and HIV among various groups. *British Journal of Addiction* 87, 1663–1668.

Rapp, R. 1987. Family and class in contemporary America. In *Rethinking the Family*, B. Thorne and M. Yalom (eds), 168–187. Boston: Northeastern University Press.

Ratliff, E. 1999. Women as 'sex workers', men as 'boyfriends': shifting identities in Philippine go-go bars and their significance in STD/AIDS control. *Anthropology and Medicine* 6(1), 79–102.

Reis, H. and P. Shaver 1988. Intimacy as an interpersonal process. In *Handbook of Personal Relationships: Theory, Research and Interventions*, S. Duck, D. Hay, S. Hobfoll, W. Ickes and B. Montgomery (eds), 367–389. Chichester: John Wiley and Sons.

Rhodes, T. 1995. Theorizing and researching 'risk': notes on the social relations of risk in heroin users' lifestyles. In *AIDS: Safety, Sexuality and Risk*, P. Aggleton, P. Davies and G. Hart (eds), 125–143. London: Taylor and Francis.

Richardson, A. and D. Bolle (eds) 1992. *Wise Before Their Time: People with AIDS and HIV Talk About Their Lives*. London: Harper Collins.

Roberts, H., S. Smith and M. Lloyd 1992. Safety as a social value: a community approach. In *Private Risks and Public Dangers, Explorations in Sociology*. S. Scott, G. Williams, S. Platt and H. Thomas (eds), 184–200. London: Avebury.

Robinson, I. 1990. Personal narratives, social careers and medical courses: analysing life strategies in autobiographies of people with multiple sclerosis. *Social Science and Medicine* 30, 1173–1186.

Robinson, P. and R. Croucher 1994. The satisfaction of men with HIV infection attending a dedicated dental clinic: a controlled study. *AIDS Care* 6, 39–48.

Ross, M. (ed) 1995. *HIV/AIDS and Sexuality*. Binghamton, NY: Harrington Park Press.

Ross, M. and C. Hunter 1991. Dimensions, content and validation of the fear of AIDS schedule in health professionals. *AIDS Care* 3, 175–180.

Roth, N.L. and M.S. Nelson 1997. HIV diagnosis rituals and identity narratives. *AIDS Care* 9, 161–180.

Rotheram-Borus, M.J., K. Mahler and M. Rosario 1995. AIDS prevention with adolescents. *AIDS Education and Prevention* 7, 320–336.

Royer, A. 1998. *Life With Chronic Illness: Social and Psychological Dimensions*. Westport, CT: Bergen and Garvey.

Rozin, P. and C. Nemeroff 1990. The laws of sympathetic magic: a psychological analysis of similarity and contagion. In *Cultural Psychology: Essays on Comparative Human Development*, J. Stigler, R. Shweder and G. Herdt (eds), 205–232. New York: Cambridge University Press.

Rymes, B. 1995. The construction of moral agency in the narratives of high-school drop-outs. *Discourse and Society* 6, 495–516.

Sacks, V. 1996. Women and AIDS: an analysis of media misrepresentations. *Social Science and Medicine* 42, 59–73.

219

BIBLIOGRAPHY

Sandstrom, K.L. 1990. Confronting deadly disease: the drama of identity construction among gay men with AIDS. *Journal of Contemporary Ethnography* 19, 271–294.

Scambler, G. 1984. Perceiving and coping with stigmatising illness. In *The Experience of Illness*, R. Fitzpatrick, J. Hinton, J. Hinton, S. Newman, G. Scambler and J. Thompson (eds), 203–226. London: Tavistock Publications.

Scambler, G and A. Hopkins 1986. Being epileptic: coming to terms with stigma. *Sociology of Health and Illness* 8, 26–43.

Schaefer, S., E. Coleman and A.M. Moore. 1995. Sexual aspects of adaptation to HIV/AIDS. In *HIV/AIDS and Sexuality*, M.W. Ross (ed), 59–72. Binghamton, NY: Harrington Press.

Schnell, D., D. Higgins, R. Wilson, G. Goldbaum, D. Cohn and R. Wolitski. 1992. Men's disclosure of HIV test results to male primary sex partners. *American Journal of Public Health* 82, 1675–1676.

Schwartz, T. 1978. Where is the culture? Personality as the distributive locus of culture. In *The Making of Psychological Anthropology*, G. Spindler (ed), 419–441. Berkeley: University of California Press.

Schwarzer, R. and Leppin, A. 1988. Social support and health: a meta-analysis. *Psychology and Health* 2, 1–15.

Scneider, J. and P. Conrad 1981. Medical and sociological typologies: the case of epilepsy. *Social Science and Medicine* 15(a), 211–219.

Scottish Council Foundation 1998. *Three Nations: Social Exclusion in Scotland.* Paper 3. (Report published on Website www.scottishpolicy.net.org.uk). Accessed April 1999.

Scully, C. and P. Mortimer 1994. Gnashings of HIV. *Lancet* 334, 904.

Shedlin, M. and J. Schreiber 1994. *Using Focus Groups in Drug Abuse and HIV/AIDS Research.* Paper prepared for the National Institute on Drug Abuse (NIDA) Technical Review: Qualitative Methods in Drug Abuse and HIV Research, Washington DC, July.

Sherr, L. 1991. *HIV and AIDS in mothers and babies: a guide to counselling.* Oxford: Blackwell Scientific Publications.

Shtarkshall, R. and T. Awerbuch 1992. It takes two to tango but one to infect. *Journal of Sex and Marital Therapy* 18, 121–127.

Siegel, K. and B. Krauss 1991. Living with HIV infection: adaptive tasks of seropositive gay men. *Journal of Health and Social Behaviour* 32, 17–32.

Simoni, J.M., H.R. Mason, G. Marks, M.S. Ruiz, D. Reed and J.L. Richardson 1995. Women's self-disclosure of HIV infection: rates, reasons, and reactions. *Journal of Consulting Clinical Psychology* 63, 474–478.

Singer, M. (ed) 1998. *The Political Economy of AIDS.* Amityville, NY: Baywood Publishing.

Singer, M. 1999. Anthropology and the politics of AIDS fatigue. *Anthropology Newsletter* 40(3), 58.

Singer, M., F. Valentin, H. Gaer and Z. Jia 1992. Why does Juan Garcia have a drinking problem: the perspective of critical medical anthropology. *Medical Anthropology* 14, 77–108.

Sobo, E.J. 1987. Geisha: institutionalization and transformation. MA thesis, University of California at San Diego.

Sobo, E.J. 1993a. Inner-city women and AIDS: the psycho-social benefits of unsafe sex. *Culture, Medicine, and Psychiatry* 17, 455–485.

Sobo, E.J. 1993b. *One Blood: The Jamaican Body.* Albany: State University of New York Press.

Sobo, E.J. 1994. Attitudes toward HIV testing among inner-city women. *Medical Anthropology* 16, 17–38.

Sobo, E.J. 1995a. Self-disclosure of positive HIV serostatus to sexual partners in the southwestern USA: a preliminary project. Paper presented to the University of Durham Department of Anthropology Seminar Series, January.

Sobo, E.J. 1995b. *Choosing Unsafe Sex: AIDS-Risk Denial among Disadvantaged Women.* Philadelphia: University of Pennsylvania Press.

Sobo, E.J. 1997. Self-disclosure and self-construction among HIV-positive people. the rhetorical uses of stereotypes and sex. *Anthropology and Medicine* 4, 67–87.

Sobo, E.J. 1999. Cultural models and HIV/AIDS: new anthropological views. *Anthropology and Medicine* 6(1), 5–12.

Sobo, E.J., G. Zimet, T. Zimmerman and H. Cecil 1997. Doubting the experts: AIDS misconceptions among runaway adolescents. *Human Organization* 56, 311–320.

Solomon, M. and W. DeJong 1989. Preventing AIDS and other STDs through condom promotion: a patient education intervention. *American Journal of Public Health* 79, 453–458.

Sontag, S. 1991. *Illness as Metaphor and AIDS and its Metaphors.* London: Penguin Books.

Stall, R. 1997. Trends in sexual risk-taking in San Francisco. Paper presented to the Safer Communities conference, Los Angeles County Department of Health, Los Angeles, April 1.

Stanley, L.D. 1999. Transforming AIDS: the moral management of a stigmatized identity. *Anthropology and Medicine* 6, 103–120.

Stein, M.D., K.A. Freedberg, L.M. Sullivan, J. Savetsky, S.M. Levenson, R. Hingson and J.H. Brown 1998. Sexual ethics: disclosure of HIV-positive status to partners. *Archives of Internal Medicine* 158, 253–257.

Strauss, C. 1992. Models and Motives. In *Human Motives and Cultural Models*, R. D'Andrade and C. Strauss (eds), 1–20. New York: Cambridge University Press.

Strauss, R.P., I.B. Corless, J.W. Lucky, C.M. v.d. Horst and B.H. Dennis 1992. The validity of self-reported HIV antibody test results. *American Journal of Public Health* 82, 567–569.

Sutherland, E. 1940. White collar criminality. *American Sociological Review* 5, 1–12.

Taerk, G., R. Gallop, W. Lancee, R. Coates and M. Fanning 1993. Recurrent themes of concern in groups for health care professionals. *AIDS Care* 5, 215–222.

Taylor, C. and D. Lourea. 1992. HIV prevention: a dramaturgical analysis and practical guide to creating safer sex interventions. In *Rethinking AIDS Prevention*, R. Bolton and M. Singer (eds), 105–146. New York: Gordon and Breach Science Publishers.

Toft, B. 1996. Limits to the mathematical modelling of disasters. In *Accident and Design: Contemporary Debates in Risk Management*, C. Hood and D.K.C. Jones (eds), 99–110. London: University College London Press.

BIBLIOGRAPHY

Travers, M. and L. Bennet 1996. AIDS, women and power. In *AIDS as a Gender Issue: Psychosocial Perspectives*, L. Sherr, C. Hankins and L. Bennett (eds), 64–77. London: Taylor and Francis.

Treichler, P. 1987. AIDS, homophobia, and biomedical discourse: an epidemic of signification. *Cultural Studies* 1, 263–305.

Treichler, P. 1992. AIDS, HIV, and the cultural construction of reality. In *The Time of AIDS: Social Analysis, Theory, and Method*, G. Herdt and S. Lindenbaum (eds), 65–98. Newbury Park, CA: Sage Publications.

Treichler, P. 1993. AIDS, gender, and biomedical discourse: current contests for meaning. In *American Feminist Thought at Century's End: A Reader*, L. Kaufman (ed), 281–384. Cambridge: Blackwell.

Turner, H., R. Hays and T. Coates 1993. Determinants of social support among gay men: the context of AIDS. *Journal of Health and Social Behavior* 34, 37–53.

Turner, P. 1993. *I Heard It Through the Grapevine: Rumor in African-American Culture*. Los Angeles: University of California Press.

Turner, R.J. and F. Marino 1994. Social support and social structure: a descriptive epidemiology. *Journal of Health and Social Behavior* 35, 193–212.

Valdiserri, R., V. Arena, D. Proctor and F. Bonati 1989. The Relationship between Women's Attitudes about Condoms and Their Use: Implications for Condom Promotion Programs. *American Journal of Public Health* 79, 499–501.

Välimäki, M., T. Suominen and I. Peate 1998. Attitudes of professionals, students and the general public to HIV/AIDS and people with HIV/AIDS: A review of the research. *Journal of Advanced Nursing* 27, 752–759.

Van Der Straten, A., K.A. Vernon, K.R. Knight, C.A. Gomez and N.S. Padian 1998. Managing HIV among serodiscordant heterosexual couples: serostatus, stigma and sex. *AIDS Care* 10, 533–548.

Vander Linden, C. 1993. NIMH prevention research helps women change AIDS risk behavior. *Public Health Reports* 3, 413.

VanLandingham, M., J. Knodel, C. Saengtienchai and A. Pramualratana 1994. Aren't sexual issues supposed to be sensitive? *Health Transition Review* 4, 85–90.

Wadsworth, E. and K. McCann 1992. Attitudes towards and use of general practitioner services among homosexual men with HIV infection or AIDS. *British Journal of General Practice* 42, 107–110.

Waldby, C., S. Kippax and J. Crawford. 1995. HIV-related discrimination in medical teaching texts. In *AIDS: Safety, Sexuality and Risk*, P. Aggleton, P. Davies and G. Hart (eds), 20–36. London: Taylor and Francis.

Walker, R. 1991. *AIDS Today, Tomorrow: an Introduction to the HIV Epidemic in America*. New Jersey: Humanities Press International.

Wang, C. 1993. Culture, meaning and disability: injury prevention campaigns and the production of stigma. In *Perspectives on Disability*, M. Nagler (ed), 77–90. Palo Alto, CA: Health Markets Research.

Ward, M. 1993a. A different disease: AIDS and health care for women in poverty. *Culture, Medicine, and Psychiatry* 17, 413–430.

Ward, M. 1993b. Poor and positive: two contrasting views from inside the AIDS epidemic. *Practicing Anthropology* 15, 59–61.

Watney, S. 1994. *Practices of Freedom: Selected Writings on HIV/AIDS.* Durham, NC: Duke University Press.

Weatherburn, P., P.M. Davies, F. Hickson, A.P.M. Coxon and T.J. McManus 1993. Sexual behaviour among HIV antibody positive gay men. Poster (PO-D20-3996) presented at IXth International Conference on AIDS, Berlin.

Weatherburn, P., A.J. Hunt, P.M. Davies, A.P.M. Coxon and T.J. McManus 1991. Condom use in a large cohort of homosexually active men in England and Wales. *AIDS Care* 3, 31–41.

Webster, N. (ed) 1983. *Webster's New Twentieth Century Dictionary of the English Language, Unabridged.* New York: Simon and Schuster.

Weinstein, N. 1984. Why it won't happen to me: perceptions of risk factors and susceptibility. *Health Psychology* 3, 431–457.

Weinstein, N. 1987. Unrealistic optimism about susceptibility to health problems: conclusions from a community-wide sample. *Journal of Behavioral Medicine* 10, 481–500.

Weinstein, N. 1989. Perceptions of personal susceptibility to harm. In *Primary Prevention of AIDS: Psychological Approaches,* V. Mays, G. Albee and S. Schneider (eds), 142–167. Newbury Park, CA: Sage Publications.

Weitz, R. 1989. Uncertainty and the lives of persons with AIDS. *Journal of Health and Social Behaviour* 30, 270–281.

Wellings, K. and J. Wadsworth 1990. AIDS and the moral climate. In *British Social Attitudes the 7th report,* R. Jowell, S. Witherspoon and L. Brook (eds), 109–126. Aldershot: Gower Publishing Company.

West, P. 1979. *An Investigation Into the Social Construction and Consequences of theLabel Epilepsy.* PhD Thesis, Bristol University.

Weyant, R., M. Bennett, M. Simon and J. Palaisa 1994. Desire to treat HIV-infected patients: similarities and differences across health-care professions. *AIDS* 8, 117–121.

White, D., K. Phillips, G. Mulleady and C. Cupitt 1993. Sexual issues and condom use among injecting drug users. *AIDS Care* 5, 381–391.

WHO [World Health Organization] 1994. *The Current Global Situation of the HIV/AIDS Pandemic.* World Health Organization, 4 January.

WHO [World Health Organization] 1998. *HIV/AIDS and Sexually Transmitted Diseases Newsletter (Dec '97 – Mar '98).* World Health Organization, Office of HIV/AIDS and Sexually Transmitted Diseases.

Wiener, C. 1975. The burden of rheumatoid arthritis: tolerating the uncertainty. *Social Science and Medicine* 9, 97–104.

Wilkie, P., I. Markova, S. Naji and C. Forbes 1990. Daily living problems of people with haemophilia and HIV infection: implications for counselling. *International Journal of Rehabilitation Research* 13, 15–25.

BIBLIOGRAPHY

Williams, B. 1994. Patient satisfaction: a valid concept? *Social Science and Medicine* 38, 509–16.

Williams, G. 1984. The genesis of chronic illness: narrative reconstruction. *Sociology of Health and Illness* 6, 174–200.

Williams, S. 1987. Goffman, interactionism, and the management of stigma in everyday life. In *Sociological Theory and Medical Sociology*, G. Scambler (ed), 136–164. London: Tavistock Publications.

Wolcott, D.L., S. Namir, F.I. Fawzy, M.S. Gottlieb and R.T. Mitsuyasu 1986. Illness concerns, attitudes towards homosexuality, and social support in gay men with AIDS. *General Hospital Psychiatry* 8, 395–403.

Wolitski, R.J., C.A.M. Reitmeijer, G.M. Goldbaum and R.M. Wilson 1998. HIV serostatus disclosure among gay and bisexual men in four American cities: general patterns and relation to sexual practices. *AIDS Care* 10, 599–610.

Wortman, C. 1984. Social support and the cancer patient: conceptual and methodological issues. *Cancer* 53(suppl.), 2339–2359.

Zich, J. and L. Temoshok 1987. Perceptions of social support in men with AIDS and ARC: relationships with distress and hardiness. *Journal of Applied Social Psychology* 17, 193–215.

Zola, I. 1993. Self, identity and the naming question: reflections on the language of disability. *Social Science and Medicine* 36, 167–173.

Index

225

INDEX

INDEX

INDEX

Strauss, A. 2, 57, 70, 71
Strauss, R.P. 60
stress 172
subjective side of AIDS 10–12
suicidal tendencies 63, 65, 66, 68, 111
support 96
  see also family; friends; social support
Sutherland, E. 81
symbolic capital 74

T-tests 51
Taerk, G. 121
Taylor, C. 198
telos 21–2
Temoshok, L. 50
Thomson, K. 182
Toft, B. 34
Tolle, S. 146
transmission routes 57, 128
travel restrictions 27, 42
Travers, M. 177
Treichler, P. 10, 22
trust 86, 99–100, 167
Turner, P. 24, 25
Turner, R.J. 182

unemployment 49
United Kingdom 1–2, 4, 66, 78, 121, 136,
    137, 196, 198
  Health Education Authority 27, 195
  risk landscapes 32, 33, 41
  stigma 16, 21, 22, 27, 28
  see also North-East England; Scotland
United States 1–2, 4, 5, 93, 121, 183, 196,
    198
  Centers for Disease Control and
    Prevention (CDC) 1, 64
  coping with HIV status 62, 65, 66, 71,
    78, 81
  disclosure in sexual settings 136, 137,
    138, 139–40, 157
  National AIDS Behavioural Survey 62

risk landscape 32, 33, 41, 43
stigma 11, 17–18, 20, 21, 22, 27, 28
  see also New Mexico
unsafe sex 156, 166, 167, 168
'untouchables' 75–6
urban legends 24–6

Valdiserri, R. 198
Välimäki, M. 27
Vander Linden, C. 198
VanLandingham, M. 53, 139, 1908
victim blaming 19–21
victimization 189

Wadsworth, E. 122, 199
Wadsworth, J. 27, 187
Waldby, C. 23
Wang, C. 197
Ward, M. 2, 21, 58, 73, 176, 181
Watney, S. 19, 22, 23, 24
Watson, J. 5
Weatherburn, P. 167
Webster, N. 13
Weinstein, N. 19, 156, 158
Weitz, R. 71
Wellings, K. 27, 187
Weyant, R. 121–2
White, D. 167
Wiener, C. 71
Wildavsky, A. 36
Wilkie, P. 183
Williams, B. 132
Williams, G. 58
Williams, S. 15, 197
Wilson, P. 42
Wisdom Narratives 21
Wolcott, D.L. 183
Wolitski, R.J. 43, 140–1
Wortman, C. 51, 182

Zich, J. 50
Zola, I. 13, 15